Authors' Disclaimer: The advice in the following chapters and supplemental materials is not intended to take the place of a physician's recommendations regarding medications or a prescribed treatment plan. Consult with your doctor about any changes you desire to make as a result of reading this book.

Published by M. Evans
An imprint of The Rowman & Littlefield Publishing Group, Inc.
4501 Forbes Boulevard, Suite 200, Lanham, Maryland 20706
http://www.rlpgtrade.com

Estover Road, Plymouth PL6 7PY, United Kingdom

Distributed by National Book Network

British Library Cataloguing in Publication Information Available

Library of Congress Cataloging-in-Publication Data

Rhoden, Chad A., 1976–
  Bringing down high blood pressure / Chad A. Rhoden, with Sarah Wiley Schein.
    p. cm.
  Includes index.
  ISBN 978-1-59077-159-4 (cloth : alk. paper) — ISBN 978-1-59077-160-0 (electronic)
  1. Hypertension—Diet therapy. 2. Salt-free diet. 3. Hypertension—Exercise therapy. I. Schein, Sarah Wiley, 1977– II. Title.
  RC685.H8R446 2010
  616.1'3206—dc22

                                                                                              2009049944

∞ ™ The paper used in this publication meets the minimum requirements of American National Standard for Information Sciences—Permanence of Paper for Printed Library Materials, ANSI/NISO Z39.48-1992.

Printed in the United States of America

BRINGING DOWN HIGH BLOOD PRESSURE

CHAD A. RHODEN, M.D., PH.D.
with Sarah Wiley Schein, M.S., R.D., L.D.N.

M. Evans

Lanham · New York · Boulder · Toronto · Plymouth, UK

BRINGING DOWN HIGH BLOOD PRESSURE

To my late grandmothers, Amy Jean Rhoden and Golia Williams,
for all of their wisdom, guidance, and unconditional love.

"Above all things that you may prosper and be in good health."
—3 John 1:2

CONTENTS

Contents

ACKNOWLEDGMENTS

FIRST AND FOREMOST, I give my humble thanks to our generous God and our Savior Jesus Christ for making this book and anything else a reality.

Next, my love and appreciation go to my beautiful, loving wife, Rhonda, for her patience with me in the publication process and her lifetime commitment to and support of our family. Of course, I am also blessed to have my wonderful children Luke Allen and Briley Belle and the perseverance they naturally provide in me daily.

For the unconditional love from both of my parents.

To our family at Broadmoor Baptist Church for the positive surroundings, Christian brotherhood, and influence in my life.

Also, I would certainly like to thank Kristin Johnson for her unselfish editorial work on this book, David Leonhardt, and all of the great staff at our publisher M. Evans for all of their commitment to making this book a success.

Chapter 1

WHAT IS HIGH BLOOD PRESSURE AND WHY IS IT IMPORTANT?

Blood Pressure 101

BLOOD PRESSURE is the pressure acting on blood vessel walls when blood flows through the arteries. Blood vessels act as pipelines for blood and transport it from the pumping heart to body tissues and organs. Every time the heart beats, blood is pumped out of the heart, which causes the pressure to increase. Between heartbeats, when the heart is at rest, the heart refills with blood and the pressure in the arteries drops.

Problems arise when the heart fills up again, but the pressure in the arteries stays at the same level or even rises. This creates excess tension in the arteries and stresses arterial walls. This tension is known as high blood pressure. Blood pressure depends on two factors: the cardiac output, or the volume of blood pumped out of the heart, and the peripheral resistance of the body's blood vessels to the flow of blood throughout the circulatory system.

Think of the circulatory system as a garden hose. In a garden hose, the water pressure can be increased by opening the faucet to allow a greater volume of water or by tightening the nozzle to narrow the spray, which increases the resistance to the flow of water. The circulatory system functions the same way. The total volume of blood the heart pumps out is affected by the total fluid volume in the blood vessels, as well as the rate and effectiveness of the heart's pumping. The size of the small arteries affects the pressure in the system. These small arteries have muscle fibers in their walls that can cause them to constrict or dilate, regulating the flow of blood in the "pipe network." If you cut off part of the hose, the volume of water builds up to extreme levels, and there is increased resistance. This is when high blood pressure can result in sudden and often fatal heart attacks and strokes.

Your body contains thousands of miles of blood vessels besides arteries and arterioles that feed your heart, brain, and other organs. When a vessel gets clogged and/or a clot breaks free and travels to your heart or brain, a heart attack or stroke can result. High blood pressure hinders your circulation, which weakens your body and your ability to resist the development of heart disease. Because of this excess stress, high blood pressure triples your risk of death from a heart attack and increases the risk of stroke by sevenfold! This makes checking your high blood pressure as important as stepping on the scale or taking your temperature.

Measuring High Blood Pressure

Blood pressure, which is measured using mercury, is made up of two forces in the arteries: systolic pressure and diastolic pressure. The top number corresponds to the systolic pressure produced as the heart contracts. The second number refers to the diastolic pressure produced when the heart relaxes between beats. The overall blood pressure reading is the top number over the bottom number (systolic/diastolic). For an adult, a blood pressure no greater than 120/80 mmHg is considered optimal. A blood pressure between 120/80 mmHg and 130/85 mmHg is considered normal, and values between 130/85 mmHg and 139/89 mmHg are considered high normal. Severe and dangerously high blood pressure is defined as systolic blood pressure equal to or greater than 180 mmHg and diastolic blood pressure equal to or greater than 120 mmHg.

The American Heart Association and the National Heart, Lung and Blood Institute (NHLBI) define high blood pressure as one or both of two things:

- Systolic pressure of 140 millimeters of mercury or higher and/or diastolic pressure of 90 millimeters of mercury or higher.
- Taking medicine to lower blood pressure.

Individual blood pressure can vary especially when patients are nervous or excited during a doctor visit. The classification of blood pressure in adults is based on the average of two or more properly measured, seated blood pressure readings on each of two or more office visits. Studies suggest ambulatory blood pressure measurement, which provides a measure of the average blood pressure over 24 hours, may be a better predictor of clinical high blood pressure.

Prehypertension or pre–high blood pressure is an American classification for when blood pressure is elevated above normal but not to the level considered to be hypertension (high blood pressure). The seventh report of the Joint National Committee (JNC 7) proposed a new definition of blood pressure values below 140/90 mmHg. Pre–high blood pressure is considered to be blood pressure readings with a systolic pressure from 120 to 139 mmHg or a diastolic pressure from 80 to 89 mmHg. Readings greater than or equal to 140/90 mmHg are considered high blood pressure.

The definition of high blood pressure has changed over the years. We now know individuals who maintain blood pressures at the low end of these numbers have much better long-term cardiovascular health. When the systolic and diastolic pressures fall in different ranges, the value of the higher range is used to classify a person as having high blood pressure or normal blood pressure. Rises in diastolic blood pressure were previously regarded as a more important risk factor than systolic elevations, but now it seems that systolic high blood pressure represents a greater risk.

Doctors debate the aggressiveness and relative value of methods used to lower pressures into the normal range for those who don't maintain such pressure on their own.

Treatment of high blood pressure is very important so that numbers don't skyrocket to dangerous levels that may precipitate strokes, heart attacks, and aortic aneurysms.

JoAnn's Story

When persistent chest pains prompted a visit to the emergency room, JoAnn had to cancel another out-of-town business trip and undergo a series of medical tests and lab work to determine the cause of her chest pain. She had gained over 100 pounds above her normal weight from eating rich foods at home and while traveling on business. She rarely exercised and was behind on her yearly medical checkup despite feeling poorly for several months.

JoAnn had to admit her once-exciting work was no longer fun, and she now dreaded going to work. Pressure from tight deadlines and irritating coworkers added to her stress.

Lying on a gurney in the ER, JoAnn feared the worst, and her mind rushed over potential outcomes and how long she'd be off work. She wondered if the launch of several consumer products would have to be postponed.

After a heart stress test and a series of additional tests, JoAnn was found to have elevated blood pressure of 155/95 mmHg readings, diabetes, elevated liver enzymes, enlarged liver with fatty deposits, significant abdominal fat, joint pain, gastric reflux, and acute anxiety, which brought on her chest pain. Her heart was healthy, but her cholesterol was elevated at 230 milligrams/deciliter (mg/dl).

JoAnn had all the risk factors for high blood pressure (and metabolic syndrome) as a result of weight gain and a sedentary lifestyle. These findings suggest JoAnn should:

- Lose weight using a low-fat, low-sodium, and moderate carbohydrate diet.
- Work with her doctor on medications for high blood pressure, elevated cholesterol, and diabetes.
- Attend a seminar on diabetes management.
- Walk a few blocks at a time and build up to at least one mile every day.
- Reduce stress through meditation or relaxation techniques and consider less-stressful job opportunities.
- Eat more fish rich in omega-3 fatty acids instead of red meat.
- Substitute low-sodium, light, or fat-free dressings for regular salad dressings.
- Drink 64 ounces of water per day.
- Develop a list of her favorite healthy foods.
- Learn to shop for and eat low glycemic index foods to better manage blood sugar.
- Increase daily intake of fruits and vegetables.
- Reduce her consumption of fruit juice to four ounces daily and eat whole fruits instead.
- Reduce her salt intake and look for low-sodium products when shopping.

Now two years later and 65 pounds lighter, JoAnn has blood pressure readings averaging 110/70 mmHg. She still needs to lose weight but is close to being able to eliminate her blood pressure medication. She credits her daily walks, diet changes, and her career change as principal factors in reducing her high blood pressure.

Dangers of Severe High Blood Pressure

According to the Seventh Report of the Joint National Committee on Prevention, Detection, Evaluation, and Treatment of High Blood Pressure (the JNC 7 report), severe high blood pressure can produce a variety of acute, life-threatening complications, which are considered high blood pressure emergencies. These include high blood pressure encephalopathy (which literally means *disease of the brain*), bleeding or swelling in the eye, and acute kidney failure. Terminology describing high blood pressure emergencies can be confusing—high blood pressure crisis, malignant high blood pressure, high blood pressure urgency, and accelerated high blood pressure are all used. The diagnosis of a high blood pressure emergency is not only based on the absolute level of blood pressure, but also on an individual's prior regular level of blood pressure. These emergencies seem to occur most commonly among patients who have not been diagnosed or have not followed a prescribed medication regimen. However, severe high blood pressure can also occur in those who take medications as directed. In case of a high blood pressure emergency, the blood pressure should be lowered slowly with one or more medications. It is important not to lower blood pressure too abruptly, as rapid reductions in blood pressure may precipitate damage to the heart, brain, or kidneys.

Measuring Your Blood Pressure at Home

Home blood pressure readings can vary from measurements taken in the traditional doctor's office and hospital environment. Home readings, however, can be helpful in evaluating symptoms suggestive of high blood pressure because these symptoms aren't often present during the few minutes of a typical physician's office visit. In fact, home monitoring can be a useful part of high blood pressure treatment.

Individuals who measure blood pressure at home have an advantage, since their focus is on monitoring the condition. True blood pressure may even be more accurately assessed by a series of home readings than by one or two "casual" office blood pressure (BP) measurements. Home readings can be a useful adjunct to information obtained in the physician's office, especially when the two are widely disparate. Long-term studies have shown that people with much lower home BP readings suffer fewer major cardiovascular events than do people who have elevated readings both in the office and at home. The same techniques used in doctors' offices should be used when measuring blood pressure at home. Sit quietly for two to five minutes first and make sure the "bladder" of the blood pressure cuff covers 80 percent of the circumference of the arm. Make sure you sit comfortably and rest your arm in the cuff parallel with your heart and your palm up.

Individuals with high blood pressure should keep an ongoing record of the blood pressure measurements and the time and date they are taken to share with their doctor at the next appointment. Any device used at home should pass Aggressive Standards for Advancement of Medical Instruments. If home readings are taken, the home measuring device should be calibrated against a standard sphygmomanometer.

I recommend the following devices for measuring blood pressure at home:

- Omron (http://www.omronhealthcare.com)
- Microlife (http://www.microlifeusa.com)
- A&D Medical Lifesource (http://www.lifesourceonline.com)

People who have been diagnosed with dangerously high blood pressure may benefit from measuring blood pressure daily as a proactive step to managing high blood pressure. You will be encouraged by the effects of exercise and diet changes. If you are on medication, this will also help you assess how well your medication is controlling your blood pressure.

What Causes High Blood Pressure?

In many cases, the exact cause of the high blood pressure is difficult to determine. This "unspecified-cause" blood pressure is known as essential high blood pressure or primary high blood pressure. That may seem a little confusing until you think of it as something that is inherently characteristic. Individuals have their own physiological and genetic makeup. Inherent and unchangeable characteristics include:

- **Heredity:** Individuals are at increased risk if one or both of their parents have high blood pressure.
- **Gender:** Men are at slightly higher risk than women, but high blood pressure in women often goes undiagnosed and untreated.
- **Age:** The risk of developing high blood pressure increases with age.
- **Race:** African Americans are at higher risk.

Let's look at the influences of gender, age, and race in more detail.

Gender

Are you more likely to have high blood pressure if you are XX (female) or if you are XY (male)? This is a question many patients ask, and the picture is somewhat mixed. We know that for the most part, men and women have the same risks for high blood pressure. However, men may be more likely to develop high blood pressure before age 55.

Age

Getting older does not reduce the need to treat high blood pressure. On the contrary, as people age, all the same health problems are present, but many related risks, such as the risk of high blood pressure, increase. As people grow older, their arteries get stiffer and blood pressures naturally tend to increase. There are many benefits of lowering elevated systolic blood pressure in seniors, and clinical studies show enormous benefits of controlling high blood pressure in the later years of life. Healthy aging is a beautiful process, and recent studies suggest seniors who adopt a healthy lifestyle experience a reduction in high blood pressure and chronic conditions such as heart disease or stroke.

Census Bureau projections suggest the number of Americans over 65 will be well over 100 million by the year 2050. Given these figures, there is a need to redouble efforts to help senior Americans manage high blood pressure and related diseases.

Race

The prevalence of high blood pressure in African Americans is among the highest in the world. This means that a greater percentage of African Americans have high blood pressure than the majority of other ethnic groups. In addition, there is a relatively lower rate of diagnosis and treatment of high blood pressure among African Americans.

Compared with Caucasians, African Americans develop high blood pressure earlier in life, and average blood pressures are much higher in African Americans. In adult African Americans, the total prevalence of high blood pressure is slightly higher than in Caucasians (28.1 percent versus 23.2 percent). However, high blood pressure is much more common among young adult African Americans, particularly young women. For example, in the 35 to 44 age range, high blood pressure occurs in 8.5 percent of white women and 22.9 percent of African American women. One-third of all African American women suffer from high blood pressure.

African Americans, like all groups, often do not receive treatment until blood pressure has been elevated a long time and major organ damage is present. The African American population has a higher incidence of high blood pressure–related illness and death, including end-stage kidney disease. African Americans have an 80 percent higher stroke mortality rate, a 50 percent higher heart disease mortality rate, and a greater than 300 percent rate of high blood pressure–related end-stage renal disease than seen in the general population. When compared with Caucasians, African Americans receiving adequate treatment will achieve similar overall declines in blood pressure and may experience a lower incidence of cardiovascular disease.

Although African Americans seem to struggle most with this condition, it also significantly affects other ethnicities. Heart disease is the leading cause of death for all races, and there is a strong association between high blood pressure and heart disease.

The rate of blood pressure control among Hispanics in the United States is less than in Caucasians *and* African Americans. Asian-American/Pacific Islander women have much lower blood pressure screening rates than other minority women, although high blood pressure is a significant problem for these women. This is the opposite in Native Americans and Alaska Natives. In a recent survey published by the Centers for Disease Control, survey respondents answered the question, "Have you ever been told by a doctor, nurse, or other health professional that you have high blood pressure?" The survey found that the high blood pressure prevalence in Native Americans/Alaska Natives is higher than the national average. Certainly all ethnic groups should pay close attention to blood pressure.

Generally, when we talk about high blood pressure related to ethnicity, we refer to essential high blood pressure, as mentioned previously. A better word to describe essential high blood pressure is **primary** high blood pressure, which, genetic factors aside, indicates that no specific medical cause can be found to explain a patient's condition. We can distinguish between primary high blood pressure and secondary high blood pressure.

Think of it this way: When something goes wrong in one part of your body, a ripple effect can create problems like high blood pressure. In secondary high blood pressure, the condition of high blood pressure is a result of, or secondary to, another condition, such as diabetes mellitus, certain kinds of tumors, and kidney disease. In fact, 5 to 10 percent of high blood pressure cases are caused by an underlying condition, according to the American Heart Association. Secondary high blood pressure tends to appear suddenly. But the good news is that proper treatment can often control or cure both the underlying condition and the high blood pressure. Although there may not always be an obvious cause for high blood pressure, controlling high blood pressure reduces the risk of serious complications, including heart disease, stroke, and kidney failure.

Another piece of the puzzle is that a variety of risk factors can complicate or bring about high blood pressure. These are lifestyle choices and/or environmental factors.

- **Alcohol:** Heavy drinking increases blood pressure.
- **Weight:** The more overweight you are, the greater your chances of developing high blood pressure.
- **Smoking:** Nicotine shrinks small blood vessels, which increases blood pressure.
- **Contraceptive and hormone use:** Blood pressure increases in women who are on the Pill or use contraceptive patches or NuvaRing, especially if women also drink alcohol and smoke cigarettes.
- **Sodium consumption:** Some people are sensitive to sodium content in their food or beverages. The risk of high blood

pressure increases when salt-sensitive people eat any form of salt. This is especially true of African Americans. Salt sensitivity is present in 45 to 50 percent of all people with high blood pressure.

- **Sedentary lifestyle:** Lack of regular exercise means that the heart works less efficiently and blood vessels have less tone and flexibility.
- **Pregnancy:** Extra blood flow and weight gain in pregnancy can increase blood pressure in women, especially ones with a family history of high blood pressure, even if blood pressure was consistently normal before the pregnancy.
- **Repressed anger and unmanaged stress:** Some studies show that people who don't express their anger/emotions or who have excess stress have a higher risk of high blood pressure and heart problems.
- Medications used for other conditions (e.g., decongestants) such as over-the-counter and prescription antihistamines for allergy.
- Street drug abuse can result in rapid rise in blood pressure both from drug toxicity and chemicals added to cut pure drug content. Fatal strokes have been reported in young cocaine users.

The causes of high blood pressure are less troubling than the long-term effects. If left untreated, persistent high blood pressure can lead to strokes, heart attacks, heart failure, arterial aneurysm, and kidney failure. Even moderate elevation of arterial blood pressure leads to shortened life expectancy.

Martin's Story

After losing his wife to cancer at an early age, Martin sought to alleviate his grief with alcohol. Two years later he found love again and remarried. One year into his marriage, he and his entire R&D team were laid off when the telecommunications industry suffered a significant downturn in mobile phone sales. He started with the company as a master's-degreed engineer and for 30 years he gave everything to the company. Despite enormous stress, he soldiered on through the best and worst of times.

The loss of a high-paying job Martin hoped would take him through retirement was another tragedy that left him feeling depressed and worthless. Once again, Martin sought solace in the bottle. Although Martin was aware his drinking was contributing to his high blood pressure, he made a habit of stopping drinking a week before his annual physical in hopes his blood pressure would fall to a lower level when examined. He feared medication might affect his sexual performance, and alcohol was already reducing his ability to sustain an erection. Fear of medication was his reasoning for deceiving his doctor.

Martin's blood pressure readings when he was drinking were 160/95 mmHg and becoming too troublesome to ignore. Martin's weight fluctuated between 10 and 20 pounds above his normal weight, and his parents had high cholesterol and died early of heart disease. He had been diagnosed with abnormal cholesterol 10 years earlier and was asked to take a cholesterol-lowering drug to reduce his blood cholesterol level.

This cat-and-mouse game went on for two years before Martin became ill with the flu and his blood pressure shot up to 175/105 mmHg. He had brief stroke-like symptoms, which resolved. He thought to himself, "This is God's way of giving me a second chance." He knew it was time to start taking care of himself to be a better husband to his new bride. He didn't want to have a heart attack or stroke like his parents. He finally came clean with his doctor and agreed to medication.

Martin has not been able to stop drinking, but he does take his blood pressure medication and cholesterol-lowering drug as directed by his doctor. He walks one mile twice daily and has cut back on red meat and other high-fat foods. He has also eliminated salty snacks and doesn't use salt in cooking or at the table. He now eats salads, fresh fruit and vegetables, grilled fish, and skinless chicken.

Martin's doctor has told him his chance of suffering a devastating or even fatal heart attack or stroke is greatly reduced because he takes his medication, and his chances of liver failure would decrease if he were able to stop drinking. He has lost weight and is in better physical condition as a result of his diet and exercise initiatives, and his depression has improved. His ability to maintain erections has also improved, and he is no longer fearful of sexual-performance issues while on medication. He is also considering joining Alcoholics Anonymous to help him stop drinking.

Martin's sexual-performance issues and fear of medication are all too common. Earlier medications affected sexual performance in some men. Newer blood pressure medications have reduced the risk of this side effect.

Almost every man fails to achieve an erection rigid enough for intercourse during some point in his adult life. More than 35 million American men have persistent problems achieving and maintaining an erection. The financial success of numerous erectile dysfunction drugs stems from the prevalence of this condition. These drugs help about 80 percent of men by stimulating blood flow to the penis, but for men with high blood pressure, diabetes, cardiovascular disease, and other degenerative diseases that damage nerves in the penis, these miracle drugs may not help. Difficulty getting or maintaining an erection is the result of reduced blood flow to the penis and often begins with narrowed or blocked arteries supplying blood to it. Since the arteries in the penis are small and erectile dysfunction is an easily recognized problem, this can be the first indication or symptom of high blood pressure and cardiovascular disease. Impotence can also be an early warning sign that arteries in other parts of the body are also becoming blocked with plaque that will increase the risk of heart attack and stroke.

The Number One Killer

High blood pressure is a major public health problem that will only worsen as the population ages. High blood pressure affects approximately one in four adults in the United States. Over half of Americans age 55 and older have high blood pressure, and if you are male and over 35, you are at significant risk. The lifetime probability of developing high blood pressure in the United States approaches a staggering 90 percent. At severely high pressures, defined as mean arterial pressures 50 percent or more above average, a person can expect to live no more than a few years unless the condition is appropriately treated.

Arteries bring oxygen-carrying blood to the heart muscle, and if the heart cannot get enough oxygen, chest pain, also known as angina, can occur. If the flow of blood is blocked, a heart attack results.

Jason's Story

Jason has been battling high blood pressure since having a heart attack at only 29 years old. Jason was fortunate someone at his office knew

CPR and saved his life. He was further stabilized by paramedics on the way to the ER, but the shock of a heart attack at 29 forced him to address numerous health issues. Jason was 130 pounds overweight and had blood pressure of 185/119 mmHg on admission to the ER. He had been on blood pressure medication but forgot to take it on the morning of his heart attack and hadn't visited his doctor for over a year.

After emergency bypass surgery, further clinical evaluation revealed Jason was borderline diabetic with a fasting blood sugar of 120 mg/dl and had an elevated serum cholesterol of 275 mg/dl. Most of his weight was centered in his belly, and both his parents suffered with high blood pressure and cardiovascular disease before dying in their late forties of sudden heart attacks.

Jason was worried about his health, but hadn't counted on a heart attack this early in his life. His doctor's comments about his weight and belly fat hurt his feelings, and he subsequently became disgusted with the doctor after a series of medication recommendations failed to bring down his blood pressure and control his chest pain. His stress continued to increase, and he lived in constant fear of having another heart attack at home, where there was no one to save him.

After he rejected two more doctors, a friend recommended a physician with nutrition training. The new doctor worked with Jason in a positive way and soon got his blood pressure down and lessened his chest pain considerably. His doctor recommended a dietary restriction on sugar, salt, fried foods, and red meat. He was asked to eat more salads, fresh fruit, and vegetables and limit his protein intake to three ounces of fish or chicken daily. Jason loved porterhouse steaks, pepperoni pizza, fried food, doughnuts, and rich chocolate sweets, but the threat of another heart attack gave him the motivation to change. He was also asked to exercise at a cardiac rehab center until his condition improved enough for him to safely walk alone.

Jason lost ten pounds in the two months following his surgery and felt confident he was doing the right things to control his high blood pressure and heart disease. His fears about another heart attack persisted, but they lessened as his weight and high blood pressure came down.

Now two years later, he is free of all meds and is at his recommended weight, and gets his blood pressure checked at an interval his doctor has set.

Jason's heart attack at 29 years old is more common than most people think. Heart disease kills more Americans than any other cause of death—1.5 million deaths annually. Many people don't know that cardiovascular disease claims about as many lives as the next five leading causes of death combined: cancer, chronic lower respiratory diseases, accidents, diabetes mellitus, and influenza/pneumonia. The situation is far from hopeless. For example, a mere 5 to 6 mmHg decrease in diastolic blood pressure lowers heart disease risk by 20 percent.

Many people resist doctor visits. The fear of illness or discovery of adverse health conditions is strong. In addition, people are ashamed if they haven't followed their doctor's recommendations on losing weight, consuming alcohol, or stopping smoking. Also, health insurance and managed care may make changing doctors difficult. However, don't be afraid to keep searching for a doctor who understands you as a patient and is willing to work positively with you. Your doctor will often be a family medicine doctor or internist or could be a cardiology specialist, depending on your care needs.

One important medical decision will be how often you should have a checkup or a blood pressure screening. Your physician will use your individual profile to decide on an optimal interval for your blood pressure screening. Many doctors believe semiannual visits are needed for most high blood pressure patients to confirm the adequacy of blood pressure control, maintain surveillance about weight and other modifiable risk factors, and review and renew prescriptions. A semiannual visit also allows discussion time for follow-up on lifestyle modifications and medication adjustments.

Medication is a necessary part of managing high blood pressure for many people. It's important to note that in most cases, if patients do not make long-term lifestyle modifications, medication will not be as effective in lowering high blood pressure. Your environment, diet, and intake of other substances may adversely interact with the medication. As Jason found out, the first medication he tried was not the best one for his metabolism. I'll provide an overview of blood pressure medications in Chapter 7. If you are able to make major lifestyle changes, you may be able to reduce or eliminate medication entirely. You can also reduce your risk of developing blood pressure—related diseases.

Diseases Related to High Blood Pressure

High blood pressure doesn't just cause heart disease. Increased blood pressure is the most important risk factor for stroke. Extremely high blood pressure can cause a break in a weakened blood vessel, which then bleeds in the brain and can result in a stroke. If a blood clot blocks one of the narrowed arteries, this can also cause a stroke.

Eye damage has also been linked to high blood pressure. Blood vessels in the eye can burst or bleed as a result of high blood pressure. Vision may become blurred or otherwise impaired and can result in blindness. Glaucoma has also been linked with high blood pressure.

As people age, arteries throughout the body harden, especially those in the heart, brain, and kidneys. High blood pressure is associated with these "stiffer" arteries. This, in turn, causes the heart and kidneys to work harder. As the kidneys work harder, they can become damaged, which often leads to kidney failure.

Lack of Awareness Is Deadly

Since high blood pressure is strongly linked to heart disease and to other illnesses, awareness is vital. However, according to the National Health and Nutrition Examination Survey, just over 70 percent of people who have high blood pressure are aware of it! Rates of blood pressure control are low in aware patients who are receiving treatment for high blood pressure. Ultimately, according to the survey, only 35 percent of people with high blood pressure have the condition under control.

High blood pressure is a widespread problem despite several advances and new findings that should reduce the problem, including:

- The availability of more high blood pressure medications than at any previous time in history.
- Increasing evidence to support the beneficial effects of blood pressure control.
- More clinical research about the importance of lifestyle modifications.
- More national guidelines about high blood pressure management.

There are several proposed reasons for this, and the blame does not solely rest on one individual. Health care providers, health care systems, and patients all play a role. Among health care providers, there is often a discrepancy between national guidelines and actual clinical practice in treating high blood pressure. Unfortunately, many physicians still aren't proactive in helping their patients manage blood pressure at optimum levels. To further complicate the problem, many patients don't adhere to treatment plans for high blood pressure. It is estimated that only 45 percent of high blood pressure patients practice lifestyle modifications or take medication regularly and consistently. Many patients take medication but do nothing to address the root cause of high blood pressure.

Other barriers to blood pressure control for patients are lack of access to health care and lack of health insurance. Even if people want to manage their blood pressure, some lack the resources to help them successfully do so.

The disastrous effect of not managing high blood pressure is especially apparent in selective populations. Since high blood pressure is more prevalent in older women as opposed to older men, a higher death rate from high blood pressure occurs in older women. Sixty percent of deaths attributed directly to uncontrolled high blood pressure occur in older women. Similarly, increased prevalence of high blood pressure in African Americans results in a dramatically higher incidence of fatal stroke, heart disease mortality, and kidney failure than in other racial groups.

If you have been recently diagnosed with high blood pressure or have had the condition for years, you need to manage your blood pressure to prevent life-threatening conditions from occurring. If you have taken the time to read this book, you've already won part of the battle because you are in the right mind-set and ready to learn how to bring down your blood pressure. After learning the dangers of uncontrolled blood pressure, you're likely motivated to improve your health. In the following chapters, we'll provide suggestions and guidelines on flavorful cooking without salt, weight loss, and exercise to assist you in bringing down your high blood pressure.

Chapter 2

GETTING STARTED WITH THE OPTIMUM HEALTH, EXERCISE, AND LOW-SODIUM DIET PLAN

As a nation we are dedicated to keeping physically fit
and parking as close to the stadium as possible.
—Bill Vaughan

Walking is good for solving problems.
It's like the feet are little psychiatrists.
—Pepper Giardino

Walk One Mile a Day, Add Years to Your Life

HERE'S A QUESTION FOR YOU: What can improve your mood, help relieve insomnia, and lower your risk for high blood pressure, heart disease, diabetes, and colon cancer?

The answer is consistent aerobic exercise.

Exercise is one of the most talked about, and in many ways, one of the most misunderstood ways to lower your blood pressure. Hundreds of thousands of deaths from high blood pressure–related conditions could be prevented annually through moderate physical activity. Many people think they have to make a major time commitment to fitness—lift weights an hour a day, run 10 miles a day, and go to the gym every day. Some individuals set self-defeating goals and become frustrated when they can't meet their goals. They quickly give up and return to a sedentary lifestyle. In addition, they may feel exercise won't do any good, or they can't exercise because they don't have access to the right equipment, their friends tell them exercise will put a strain on their heart, and so on. A combination of physical, psychological, social, and environmental factors influence exercise habits.

Regular exercise may take a little creativity, but it's worthwhile. Even if you just dance in a room by yourself to your favorite music on your iPod, you're getting the blood flowing and increasing circulation and flexibility throughout your whole body. No matter what your family and friends might say or think, being physically active is one of the most important steps you can take to control high blood pressure and reduce your risk of heart disease.

Dancing to those tunes on your iPod for five or ten minutes is just an example of how little effort it takes to become physically active. Dr. William Roberts once said that exercise training is "an agent with lipid-lowering, antihypertensive, positive inotropic, negative chronotropic, vasodilating, diuretic, anorexigenic, weight-reducing, cathartic, hypo-glycemic, tranquilizing, hypnotic and anti-depressive qualities."

Not everyone reading this book will recognize all of those terms, but they are all wonderful things from a medical perspective. Simply put for the purposes of this book: If you walk more often, you may reduce your blood pressure and your risk of developing heart disease.

In addition, participation in a physician-supervised cardiac reha-bilitation exercise program can prevent further heart events for patients who've had heart attacks. This is in part because of the ben-eficial effects of regular physical activity on blood pressure. In fact, by participating in an exercise program, a person decreases the chance of a subsequent deadly heart event by nearly 25 percent.

Despite the well-known benefits of physical activity, population statistics send a dismal message. Fewer than 50 percent of adults in the United States meet public health recommendations suggesting the average adult get 30 minutes of moderate activity more than five days a week. Physical activity is one of the leading health indicators designated by the Department of Health and Human Services program *Healthy People 2010* to reflect the health of the United States. Unfortunately, fewer than one in three U.S. adults engage in leisure-time active pursuits (volleyball, soccer, hiking, yoga, tennis, jogging, or swimming), and 42 percent engage in less than the recommended amount of activity. About

70 percent of adults are considered sedentary or engage in no physical activity at all! In addition, only about one-third of the adult population over 65 reports regular activity, which is a concern, considering this is the most rapidly growing segment of the U.S. population.

Overwhelming evidence suggests physical activity is a behavioral change consistently associated with improved quality of life outcomes. Former President Bill Clinton has been known as a jogger and golfer. President Clinton's case is especially noteworthy because he suffered a heart attack and has modified his lifestyle to include even more physical activity.

Get Moving and Live Longer

Regular exercise also improves your chances of living longer with a better quality of life and more stamina. No one enjoys climbing a flight of stairs and being winded! Stamina is beneficial in many situations in life and is an indicator of heart health. Exercise recommendations need to be modified to suit a person's physical condition. For example, if you've been sedentary for years or are recovering from a heart attack, you may have to build up gradually under the supervision of a person trained in CPR.

I recently spoke to a 35-year-old friend who uses the neighborhood gym often for weight lifting. Despite his years of weight lifting and a well-toned upper torso, he hasn't been following the 30-minute-a-day recommendation for aerobic activity. As a result, walking a flight of stairs leaves him short of breath! This is a scary thought to most folks and enough to encourage them toward better aerobic heart fitness. My friend had no preexisting health condition, but his body mass index (BMI) was much greater than the recommended values. The combination of increased body mass and decreased fitness has dramatically decreased his stamina and heart fitness. As a result, my friend will have to be on guard for a host of illnesses, not just heart disease and high blood pressure. Medical research now suggests consistent aerobic exercise will protect against certain types of cancer, including colon, breast, endometrial, prostate, testicular, and lung cancer.

Physicians and other health care professionals are not going to judge or ridicule you for lapses in exercise, but will aim to help you attain the best physical condition at any age.

Wesley's Story

Wesley was 55 years old when he enrolled in a blood pressure research study at our medical institution. The study objective was to investigate whether regular exercise improves blood pressure. Wesley was well over his recommended weight and had a sedentary lifestyle. In addition, his love of Italian sausage pizza added significant fat and salt to his diet. Over the last five years, his blood pressure steadily increased. The extra pounds weighed heavily on his belly. Although an athlete and avid tennis player in his youth, in his mid-forties, Wesley had back problems and did not participate in an active lifestyle.

After two months of vigorous walking during the study, Wesley's blood pressure dropped from 157/89 mmHg to 131/76 mmHg! He now plays tennis again. This real-life success story not only gives others motivation, but illustrates the value of exercise. It also shows that whether you are in your forties, sixties, or eighties, it is never too late to improve your health.

Marie's Story

Although Marie was on the high school and college swim teams, she lost interest in exercise when her children were young and she had to work part-time to make ends meet. She enjoyed walking, but usually put her family's needs first. After her children were grown and Marie retired at age 65, she simply wanted to relax. Although she and her husband bowled, Marie got out of the habit of aerobic exercise. Taking the dog out in the morning made her short of breath!

Marie ate store-bought cookies, ice cream, and salty snacks and often had difficulty concentrating and remembering, which she attributed to "old age." She smoked most of her life and quit several months before her doctor took her blood pressure, which read 160/99. Her doctor diagnosed her with high blood pressure after her readings did not change much in two more blood pressure screenings.

After learning how to control high blood pressure and following her doctor's recommendations, Marie decided to change her diet and incorporate exercise into her daily routine. Her husband supported her and bought her a pedometer—a device that measures how many steps you take and records the number of miles you walk, and can also record the number of calories burned. She set a goal of walking 10,000 to 12,000 steps a day. She huffed and puffed as she walked around the block several times with a friend in the neighborhood, but Marie kept at it. She also ate just a scoop of low-fat/low-carb ice cream for dessert and a handful of unsalted nuts in the afternoon when she most craved a sugary cookie. She didn't eliminate sweets entirely, but she cut way back!

Marie's decision became easier when Lorraine, a close friend, died suddenly of a heart attack at 65 years old. Lorraine's health history and lifestyle were nearly identical to Marie's. Her friend's sudden death was a turning point for Marie. She committed to walking one mile daily and eating whole-grain cereal with skim milk instead of her usual bacon and eggs.

Marie now feels more upbeat, has more energy and enjoys life more fully. She recently started swimming again twice a week. Now convinced, she intends to follow her blood pressure, exercise, and diet program for the rest of her life!

Watch Your Weight

Clinical research has demonstrated that extra weight causes many problems. It is a significant risk factor for a host of diseases, including diabetes, cholesterol abnormalities, heart disease, stroke, gallbladder disease, osteoarthritis, breast and colon cancer, and sleep apnea. Extra weight contributes to disabling diseases and premature death.

Excess weight ratchets up the pressure in more ways than one. Significant weight gain increases risk of high blood pressure and other related diseases. The link between high blood pressure and obesity includes sodium retention and increases in the resistance inside vessels. In other words, salt and other pressures make the blood vessels too small relative to the volume of blood passing through. Blood volume also increases with obesity, as does the amount of blood ejected from the heart.

Popular diet and exercise programs focus on losing weight to achieve the washboard abs and thin thighs we see on magazine covers. There are many benefits of exercise beyond having a great figure or looking good in a bathing suit. Exercise promotes good general health and longevity!

Losing just 5 to 10 percent of your body weight has the potential to lower your blood pressure significantly. Obesity research at the University of North Carolina School of Public Health and Medicine indicates that shedding excess pounds decreases the activity of angiotensin-converting enzyme (ACE), which is known to initiate a series of biochemical reactions that play a central role in increasing blood pressure. Blood pressure medications on the market now target this enzyme, but weight loss can mimic these effects as well. The clinical study supports prior studies that connect lower body weights with lower blood pressure and lowered risk for developing blood pressure–related organ damage.

Brief Quiz: True or False?

1. Weight reduction, as well as choosing foods lower in salt, may reduce high blood pressure.
2. Skipping meals is a good way to cut calories.
3. The best way to lose weight is to eat fewer calories and increase physical activity.

If you answered (1) true, (2) false, and (3) true, go to the head of the class. If not, read on to learn more.

Rethinking Weight Loss

If losing weight is a concern for you, you may be wondering where to start. A proposed mind-set about weight loss is an important starting point. First, **there is no magic formula for weight loss.**

Readers of this book are likely to understand that losing weight requires human beings to eat fewer calories than they burn. The number of calories an average person burns daily depends on many factors, such as level of activity, caloric intake, and body size.

Popular weight-loss fad diets often have conflicting recommendations, which makes it difficult to determine the most healthful approach to weight loss. While just about any calorie-restrictive diet will help reduce weight, long-term weight loss is rarely achieved with fad diets.

If you are overweight, you didn't accumulate the excess pounds overnight and you shouldn't expect to lose them in two weeks, no matter what the marketers of fad diets promise. Slow, steady weight loss is preferable for a variety of health reasons.

Crash diets will result in weight loss, but the weight loss is not sustainable long term. Crash diets can also be harmful to your health. Some reported/established side effects and metabolic complications for very-low-carbohydrate, high-fat/high-protein diets crash diets are:

- Coronary heart disease
- Cancer
- Type 2 diabetes
- Kidney failure
- Kidney stones
- Fatty liver and elevated liver function tests
- Cardiac arrhythmia
- Elevated serum cholesterol and triglycerides
- Elevated C-reactive protein and other inflammatory markers
- Degenerative eye disease leading to blindness
- Deficiency of important nutrients
- Gout
- Impaired cognitive function

In addition to the above potential complications, some of these diets:

- Are too low in calories.
- Don't provide adequate nourishment.
- Often result in yo-yo weight fluctuations.
- Have a significant long-term failure rate.

Losing weight and keeping it off begins with an understanding of energy intake and energy expenditure. Calories go in via the mouth and are expended through daily activity. Think of the body as a machine and calories as balls of fuel or energy. Just getting through a normal day with normal bodily functions and activities expends calories. However, if we're sedentary or sit in front of a television or a computer terminal all day long, more balls of fuel are stored. This "extra fuel" hangs around as excess pounds for weeks, months, and years. To be overweight is to be in a state of energy imbalance. We know what being overweight looks and feels like, but many of us don't understand what our ideal weight range is, or how we can attain that weight.

Body Mass Index

Two key measures are used to determine if someone is overweight: the BMI and waist circumference. (See appendix A for the formula.) BMI relates weight to height to give an approximation of total body fat, the factor that increases the risk of obesity-related diseases. Overweight is defined as a BMI of 25 to 29.9, and obesity is defined as a BMI equal to or more than 30. Currently, any person with a BMI exceeding 25 kg/m² is defined as overweight.

BMI may overestimate body fat or inaccurately estimate total body fat in muscular people or people who have lost muscle mass. For example, older people often have lost muscle mass and gained more fat than younger people. Waist measurement is often a more important indicator of overweight. Too much belly fat also increases disease risk. A waist measurement of more than 35 inches in women and more than 40 inches in men is considered a significant risk factor for heart disease and stroke.

Blossoming waist size and significant belly fat is not only a physical fitness concern, but is also a marker for predicting future health problems. These fat stores or adipose tissues secrete inflammatory proteins, which may lead to the development of cardiovascular disease, stroke, cancer, and diabetes.

In addition to cholesterol, HDL, fasting blood sugar, and triglycerides, other important markers can be identified with simple noninvasive blood testing.

- High sensitivity C-reactive protein is a marker of inflammation and has been linked to the development of cardiovascular disease and sudden death.
- Elevated fibrinogen may indicate an increased marker or risk factor for blood clots, which can travel from the point of origin to the heart, lungs, and brain and cause irreversible damage to major organs and even sudden death.

Researchers at Pennsylvania State University completed the first clinical study to show that increasing whole grain intake by consuming foods like brown rice, whole-grain barley, and oatmeal promotes not only weight loss, but decreased presence of C-reactive protein and belly fat. A control group who ate refined carbohydrates like white bread, rice, and pasta was able to lose weight, but showed no decrease in C-reactive protein and less belly fat reduction. From what we now know about the role of such "inflammatory markers," these findings certainly suggest an additional benefit of whole grains!

For people who are considered obese (BMI greater than or equal to 30), or for those who are overweight (BMI of 25 to 29.9) and have two or more heart disease risk factors, weight loss is recommended. Most people who are not overweight, do not have a high waist measurement, and have fewer than two risk factors should focus on weight maintenance rather than losing weight.

Reasonable Goals and Reasonable Portion Sizes

Often those who are overweight start out thinking they need to lose 30 pounds in 2 weeks. This is rarely attainable, and you should aim for losing no more than two pounds per week. To lose one pound of fat requires burning 3,500 calories. To put this in perspective, keep in mind that to lose one pound a week, you need to eat 500 calories less each day or burn 500 calories a day more than you usually do. Try starting with a weight loss of 10 percent of your current body weight over six months. This is the healthiest way to lose weight, and this approach offers the best chance of long-term success.

When using a diet plan for weight loss, you need to remember that there is no one diet perfect for everyone. With this in mind, a 2,000-calorie diet is reasonable for most men, and generally, a daily intake of 1,800 calories is appropriate for most women. This is, of course, a generalization. For example, a 35-year-old, 6-foot-tall male who weighs 200 pounds burns approximately 2,000 calories per day doing absolutely nothing. On the other hand, a 35-year-old, 5-foot, 6-inch female who weighs 150 pounds burns approximately 1,450 calories at rest. Therefore, a weight-loss plan should be tailored on an individual basis.

Whether your goal is weight loss or weight maintenance, I strongly recommend you strive for moderation in both weight loss and portion size. To help you understand portion control, you might want to measure portions in the beginning. You may be surprised to see how much a healthy portion is! For example, the Food Guide Pyramid recommends six to eight servings of whole grains a day, but a serving of grains equals one slice of bread or half a cup of rice or pasta. Our "supersize" culture developed from fast food advertising has given us the notion that more is better, but the calorie content of supersize portions is astonishing and contributes to excess weight. The correct portion for most proteins is 3 ounces or no larger than a deck of cards.

Even if you eat the recommended portion size, you may be tempted to scarf it down on the run. Try to eat appropriate portion sizes in a relaxed manner. Taking time to enjoy your food will reduce your calorie consumption during meals. Another useful tip is to choose lower-calorie foods that take longer to eat; for example, a large green salad over a small filet of beef.

While these suggestions make sense intellectually, they aren't the first step to losing weight. Without that first step, you may not be successful with any weight-loss program. The first step to losing weight is a simple question.

Why Do You Want to Lose Weight?

Why have you set the goal of losing weight? Most people trying to lose weight focus on just one objective: weight loss. They get caught up in that magic, elusive promise of being thin. They forget the true reasons they are losing weight: to bring down blood pressure, to manage diabetes, to feel better, and to avoid sudden heart attacks and premature death.

Opt for a different attitude toward your exercise and diet program. Envision your blood pressure and your weight being reduced to normal ranges, or at least ranges that aren't dangerously high. What an encouraging thought and excellent goal. Write down your ideal weight and blood pressure and keep these numbers on your refrigerator door, on your bathroom mirror, by the treadmill, or anywhere where you'll receive positive reinforcement.

Write down the dietary and exercise changes you desire to make to support your long-term weight-loss and blood pressure goals. Successful weight managers are those who select two or three goals at a time. Make the goals (1) specific, (2) attainable, and (3) forgivable. *Specific* means goals such as walking one mile every day or doing a 30-minute exercise DVD five days a week, rather than the vague goal of "work out more." An attainable goal is realistic. For example, make a goal to walk one mile each day, as opposed to jogging 10 miles every day. If you've been sedentary for years, check with your doctor before starting a new exercise program. *Forgivable* means not agonizing if you fail to exercise for one day or two days.

Specific and attainable goals also apply to nutritional changes. For most people, diet recommendations supported by evidence and research make tangible goals. These goals include:

- Eat five to nine servings a day of fruits and vegetables.
- Make most of your grains whole grains.
- Choose 3-ounce servings of lean protein. Balance animal and plant sources. Fish and poultry are the leanest animal proteins. Beans, nuts, and tofu are good sources of plant protein.
- Include healthy sources of fat for nutrients and satisfaction, such as nuts, nut butters, avocado, and olive and oils. Limit your sodium intake to less than 2,300 milligrams per day.

Sodium Content Alert

The table below shows the relative contribution of sodium and other nutrients in a selection of leading brands, store brands, and organic brands. All this information was collected from product labels and illustrates the large amount of sodium in a number of products.

Two important takeaways from this list are:

- Read labels carefully and select the lowest-sodium-content products available.
- Avoid high-sodium-content processed convenience foods.

A doctor friend told me that while shopping at Wal-Mart, he waited in line at the checkout and noticed a young woman with a young child who was screaming and running around the checkout area. She finished loading her groceries on the conveyor belt and said to him, "My kids insist on eating hot dogs, pizza, cookies, soda, and candy."

My friend nodded and looked at the assortment of groceries she selected. She had eight packages of hot dogs with white flour buns, five frozen pepperoni pizzas, four packages of assorted cookies, four bags of assorted miniature candy bars, and two cases of carbonated soft drinks.

Another patron behind him commented on the woman's cart once the young woman had checked out and rounded up her child. In further conversation, my friend learned that this patron had heart disease

Table 2.1. Sodium Content in Grocery Items

Food Product	Sodium	Fat	Carbohydrates	Protein	Calories per Serving
Great Value Iodized Salt	590 mg (1/4 teaspoon)	0 g	0 g	0 g	0
Great Value Harvest 9 Grain Bread	135 mg	1.5 g	14 g	3 g	80
Claussen Kosher Dill Minis	290 mg	0 g	1 g	0 g	5
Alberston's Sweet Relish	120 mg	0 g	4 g	0 g	15
Dole Pitted Dates	0 mg	0 g	30 g	<1 g	100
SunMaid Mediterranean Apricots	15 mg	0 g	23 g	1 g	100
Good Sense Cranberries 'N More Trail Mix	0 mg	10 g	13 g	4 g	150
Good Sense Cherry Cranberry Pecan Salad Pizazz Topping	10 mg	1.5 g	4 g	0 g	30
Kraft Light Catalina salad dressing	430 mg	1 g	12 g	0 g	60
Best Choice Fat-Free Italian salad dressing	450 mg	0 g	3 g	0 g	10
Kraft Mesquite Smoke Barbeque Sauce	420 mg	0 g	9 g	0 g	40
Chocolate Silk Soymilk	100 mg	3.5 g	23 g	5 g	140
The Skinny Cow Chocolate Fat-Free Milk	240 mg	0 g	26 g	11 g	150
Braum's 2 percent Reduced-Fat Milk	140 g	5 g	13	9 g	130
Braum's Extra Sharp Cheddar Cheese	180 mg	9 g	<1.0 g	7 g	110
Braum's Sweet Cream Butter	90 mg	11 g	0 g	0 g	100

Great Value Neufchatel Cream Cheese	110	6 g	2 g	2 g	70
Stouffer's Lasagna with Meat and Sauce	930 mg	11 g	38 g	24 g	350
Freschetta Ultra Thin Pepperoni Pizza	730 mg	17 g*	25 g	17 g	330
Oscar Mayer Bun–Length Wieners	680 mg	16	<1.0 g	6 g	170
Nature's Own 100 percent Whole Wheat Hot Dog Buns	190 mg	0.5 g	19 g	5 g	90
Great Value Prepared Dijon Mustard	120 mg	0 g	0 g	0	5
French's Spicy Brown Mustard	80 mg	0 g	0 g	0 g	5
Heinz Tomato Ketchup	190 mg	0	4 g	0 g	15
Frontera Chipotle Hot Sauce	35 mg	0	1 g	0 g	5
World Harbors Angostura Worcestershire Sauce	20 mg	0 g	1 g	0 g	5
Muir Glen Organic Fire Roasted Diced Tomatoes	290 mg	0	6 g	1 g	30
Campbell's Cream of Mushroom Soup	870 mg	6 g	9 g	1 g	100
Smucker's Natural Peanut Butter	120 mg	16 g	6 g	8 g	210
Target Market Pantry Old–Fashioned Oats	0 mg	2.5 g	27 g	5 g	150
Diet Coke	30 mg	0 g	0 g	0 g	0
Tropicana Valencia Orange Juice with Mango	10 mg	0 g	30 g	2 g	130
Best Choice Lite Microwave Popcorn	250 mg	5 g**	20 g	3 g	140

* (7 g saturated fat)

** (2 g trans-fat)

and slightly elevated blood pressure. You can imagine that he gave that more health-conscious patron a list of high-sodium meals to avoid:

- Salt-cured meats such as ham, bacon, sausage, salami, pepperoni, prosciutto, processed canned meat, deviled ham, corned beef, luncheon meat, hot dogs, bratwurst, chipped beef, and jerky.
- Frozen pizza and pizzas sold through major home delivery chains. Salt contributions come from crust, pepperoni, sausage, sauce, and cheese.
- Salted nuts, pretzels, crackers, potato chips, tortilla chips, corn chips, and microwave popcorn.
- Salt-cured dill pickles, okra, and olives.
- Prepared frozen entrées (except reduced-sodium varieties).
- Canned soup (except low-sodium varieties).
- Table salt added while cooking or at the table when food is served.
- Electrolyte replacement sports drinks.
- Cheeses and processed cheese products.
- Canned vegetables (except low-sodium varieties).
- Canned tomato juice, canned tomatoes, and bottled spaghetti sauce.

The Optimum Health Low-Sodium Diet

I recommend the DASH Diet (which may annoy fellow shoppers in grocery stores).

The **DASH diet** (Dietary Approaches to Stop Hypertension) is a diet promoted by the National Heart, Lung, and Blood Institute (part of the National Institutes of Health, a U.S. government organization) to control high blood pressure. A major feature of the plan is limiting intake of sodium, and it also generally encourages consumption of nuts, whole grains, fish, poultry, fruits, and vegetables while lowering consumption of red meats, sweets, and sugar. It is also "rich in potassium, magnesium, and calcium, as well as protein and fiber." Not only does the plan emphasize good eating habits, it also suggests healthy alternatives to "junk food" and discourages consumption of processed foods.

I also promote my Optimum Health Low Sodium Diet to people I speak to. Here is the Optimum Health Low Sodium Diet plan for bringing down high blood pressure:

- Use my Dr. Rhoden's FlavorDoctor heart-healthy seasoning blend, which can be found in nearby grocery stores or at www.flavordoctor.net. Also, you can visit www.shop .youroptimumhealth.net to access the link for more information.
- Cook with olive oil, canola oil, or flaxseed oil. Flaxseed oil is very high in omega-3 fatty acids. Use these oils for sautéing, in salad dressings, and for basting grilled vegetables and fish.
- Routinely eat a variety of oily fish high in omega-3 fatty acids, such as tuna, salmon, mackerel, herring, and sardines in place of meat and poultry.
- Eat whole-grain foods at every meal (oatmeal for breakfast, a whole-wheat pita sandwich for lunch, and whole-grain pasta for dinner).
- Eat dark leafy greens such as spinach, broccoli rabe, collard greens, and kale.
- When you dine out, ask waiters to provide low-sodium versions of the food you order. Ask for Dr. Rhoden's FlavorDoctor, which is found in many restaurants.
- Eat legumes such as lentils, peas, and beans. Lentil or minestrone soup is a delicious way to include legumes in your diet.
- Eat at least four whole fresh fruits every day.
- Use generous amounts of garlic and onion to flavor foods.
- Eat a handful of your favorite unsalted nuts every day.
- Limit sodium intake to less than 2,300 milligrams per day.
- If you drink, only have an occasional glass of red wine with dinner.

Americans often sacrifice healthful choices for convenience, and many convenience foods are loaded with sodium. My philosophy is to eat the right foods in moderation. A restrictive diet where all your favorite foods are forbidden will not be sustainable over the long term. In the recipe section, you'll learn to make low-calorie/fat/sugar/sodium versions of your favorite foods and dishes. Food should be enjoyed, and eating should remain a pleasurable experience.

In the next section, we'll look at micronutrients that can help lower your blood pressure, and we'll get into the nuts and bolts of eating to lower your blood pressure.

Chapter 3

EATING FOR OPTIMUM BLOOD PRESSURE

YOUR DIET PLAN to lower blood pressure emphasizes fruits, vegetables, lean proteins, and low-fat dairy foods and cuts back on portion sizes of protein-heavy foods. A diet that brings down blood pressure substitutes flavorful low-sodium marinades, rubs, relishes, salsas, vinaigrettes, and grilling seasonings for salt. In addition, your optimum blood pressure diet includes drinking red wine in moderation and having an occasional bite of dark chocolate.

There is an important relationship between good nutrition, dietary intake, and excellent health. Lifelong adoption of healthy eating habits can help you achieve optimal health and reduce the risk of sudden death from heart attack or stroke and the development of chronic debilitating diseases. We talked about sodium in the previous chapter. Unlike sodium, potassium and magnesium are micronutrients that help lower blood pressure.

Optimum Health—Micronutrients

Macronutrients are nutrients that the body normally needs in large quantities. Most vitamins and minerals fall into this category. I certainly recommend that almost everyone take a daily vitamin/mineral supplement. Since there are many options out there, it may be difficult to be confident that you have found the right one. Fruits and vegetables, however, are tasty sources of micronutrients while you choose the right vitamin/mineral supplement.

The potassium and magnesium in vegetables and fruits are micronutrients as well as electrolytes with powerful blood-pressure-lowering properties. Table 3.1 lists potassium- and magnesium-rich produce.

Table 3.1.   Potassium and Magnesium Power Foods: Fruits
and Vegetables with High Quantities

High in Potassium		High in Magnesium	
Fruits	*Vegetables*	*Fruits*	*Vegetables*
Apricots	Beets	Avocados	Artichokes
Avocados	Black-eyed peas	Bananas	Beans—black, navy,
Bananas	Brussels sprouts	Figs	white, pinto
Cantaloupes	Celery	Tomatoes	Broccoli
Dates	Garbanzo beans		Okra
Figs	Potatoes		Potatoes
Honeydews	Spinach		Soybeans
Kiwifruit	Winter squash		Spinach
Nectarines			
Oranges			
Pears			
Prunes			
Tomatoes			

A diet rich in potassium blunts the effect of salt on blood pressure. Be sure to get enough potassium in the foods you eat. Table 3.2 provides the amount of potassium in common foods.

Magnesium can similarly improve your BP readings, even though studies haven't conclusively shown that magnesium supplements or magnesium-rich foods prevent high blood pressure. It's important to maintain a healthy balance. Generally, you should get enough magnesium if you follow a healthy diet. Magnesium is found in whole grains, green leafy vegetables, nuts, and dried peas and beans. Table 3.3 shows which common foods, all of them recommended for a healthy BP-reducing diet, are high in magnesium.

Other nutrients that you need in trace amounts affect your blood pressure. Nitrates, found in vegetables such as spinach and lettuce, may

Table 3.2. Potassium Amounts in Vegetables, Fruits, and Dairy: Foods with High Quantities

Food	Serving Size	Potassium (mg)
Apricots, dried	10 halves	407
Avocados, raw	1 ounce	180
Bananas, raw	1 cup	594
Beets, cooked	1 cup	519
Brussels sprouts, cooked	1 cup	504
Cantaloupe	1 cup	494
Dates, dried	5 dates	271
Figs, dried	2 figs	271
Kiwifruit, raw	1 medium	252
Lima beans	1 cup	955
Melons, honeydew	1 cup	461
Milk, fat-free or skim	1 cup	407
Nectarines	1 nectarine	288
Orange juice	1 cup	496
Oranges	1 orange	237
Pears (fresh)	1 pear	208
Peanuts, dry roasted, without salt	1 ounce	187
Potatoes, baked, flesh and skin	1 potato	1,081
Prune juice	1 cup	707
Prunes, dried	1 cup	828
Raisins	1 cup	1,089
Spinach, cooked	1 cup	839
Tomato products, canned, sauce	1 cup	909
Winter squash	1 cup	896
Yogurt, plain, skim milk	8 ounces	579

Values were obtained from the USDA Nutrient Database for Standard References, Release 15 for Potassium (mg) content of selected foods per common measure.

http://www.nal.usda.gov/fnic/foodcomp/Data/SR15/wtrank/wt_rank.html

Table 3.3. Magnesium Amounts in Vegetables, Fruits, Fish, and Grains: Foods with High Quantities

Food	Serving Size	Magnesium (mg)
Beans, black	1 cup	120
Broccoli, raw	1 cup	22
Halibut	½ fillet	170
Nuts, peanuts	1 ounce	64
Okra, frozen	1 cup	94
Oysters	3 ounces	49
Plantain, raw	1 medium	66
Rockfish	1 fillet	51
Scallop	6 large	55
Seeds, pumpkin and squash	1 ounce (142 seeds)	151
Soy milk	1 cup	47
Spinach, cooked	1 cup	157
Tofu	¼ block	37
Whole grain cereal, ready-to-eat	¾ cup	24
Whole grain cereal, cooked	1 cup	56
Whole wheat bread	1 slice	24

Values were obtained from the USDA Nutrient Database for Standard References, Release 15 for Magnesium, Mg (mg) content of selected foods per common measure.

http://www.nal.usda.gov/fnic/foodcomp/Data/SR15/wtrank/wt_rank.html

be Mother Nature's way of keeping blood pressure in check. Nitrates in vegetables appear to keep blood vessels healthy and lower blood pressure. The *New England Journal of Medicine* reported short-term nitrate supplementation with a daily dose equivalent to the amount normally found in 150 to 250 grams of a nitrate-rich vegetable—such as spinach, lettuce, or beetroot—for three days may be associated with a lower average diastolic blood pressure (the bottom number in a blood pressure measurement) of nearly 4 mmHg! This is certainly similar to the effects seen in trials of the DASH Diet. Medical studies appear to support these findings. I certainly think it reasonable to call for more research on nitrates.

Simply consuming more potassium, magnesium, and nitrates found in vegetables as opposed to commercially sold bacon and hot dogs illustrates the power of healthy choice that you possess. Similarly, there are many more nutritional steps you can take to manage blood pressure.

Smart Shopping to Lower Your Blood Pressure

You can manage your blood pressure by having the right foods in your refrigerator and pantry. Smart shopping will make cooking and eating more enjoyable.

When you're preparing your shopping list, be wary of including your favorite fat-free products. Just because a product label reads "fat-free" doesn't mean it is calorie free or sodium free. Watching calories is as important as monitoring fat, and reduced-fat or fat-free products contain higher amounts of sodium and sugar. Label and ingredient reading will help you avoid high-sugar or high-sodium replacement products. In many cases, these foods are not healthy and you'll end up consuming as many, if not more, calories and sodium per serving than regular products.

Pay attention to serving sizes as well as servings per container and choose products that are lowest in sodium and calories per serving. As we saw in Table 2.1, light- and fat-free salad dressing can contain high sodium contributions.

Smart shopping will help you eat healthier. Fill your kitchen cupboards and refrigerator with a supply of healthy basics to make nutritious cooking easier. Here's a list of basic staples.

Leafy Greens and Fresh Produce for Salads

With the ever-increasing selection of leafy greens—such as romaine lettuce, red curly leaf lettuce, Boston Bibb lettuce, baby spinach leaves, frisee, radicchio, arugula—and ready-to-eat salad vegetables such as zucchini, bell peppers, radishes, English cucumbers, matchstick carrots, and grape tomatoes, the sky's the limit on healthy salad ingredients.

Leafy greens and salad vegetables should be included in most meals if you are trying to bring down your blood pressure and lose weight. Greens in particular are abundant in the nitrates I discussed earlier. The nitrates produce nitric oxide, which relaxes blood vessels. Vegetables in general are low density, which means that we feel full faster after we eat salad greens and zucchini as opposed to onion rings and French fries.

When you've selected your favorite greens and fresh produce, the next step is to dress these fabulous greens for maximum flavor without adding too many calories or too much salt. The marketing departments of major salad dressing companies routinely do taste testing on new product offerings. Taste preference has consistently been stronger for light salad dressings as opposed to fat-free dressings. Sodium or sugar additives are often used to improve the taste of fat-free salad dressings because of the sometimes lackluster flavor that your favorite Thousand Island variety, for example, has when void of any fat.

You'll find several healthy and excellent salad dressings in the grocery store. Organic products are increasingly more common. Additionally, a simple dressing of olive oil, lemon or balsamic vinegar, and garlic will allow you to control the sodium content. Try the low-sodium salad dressing options in the recipe section of this book.

Now that you've got the greens, fresh produce, and dressing together, remember that you can make a full meal of the salad by including three ounces of any grilled chicken, fish, or shrimp in the recipe section. Also, you can bring in black ripe olives, a sprinkling of nuts such as sunflower or pumpkins seeds, fresh fruit, or pickled beets as garnishes. Avoid adding cheese to your salad.

Fresh Produce for Grilling, Roasting, Pan Braising, Stir-Frying, or Steaming

Choose a variety of colors when selecting vegetables. Squashes, sweet potatoes, broccoli, broccolini, tomatoes, asparagus, snow peas, sugar snap peas, edamame, eggplant, beets, cabbage, kale, broccoli rabe, turnip greens, collard greens, beet greens, garlic, corn, rutabagas, turnips, parsnips, cauliflower, and red, yellow, and green onions, provide a variety of vitamins and minerals for a small number of calories.

Don't forget pumpkins! Pumpkin flesh is crammed full of phenols, a type of health-promoting antioxidant found in many plants. Pumpkin phenols in particular have many kind-to-your-body qualities and have even been thought to suppress the same enzyme as some blood pressure drugs do. Eating pumpkins therefore may theoretically reduce vascular tension and lower high blood pressure while promoting overall heart health.

Try these:

- Marinate zucchini, crookneck squash, corn, eggplant, tomatoes, bell peppers, and green and red onions with fresh or dried herbs, garlic, and olive oil and grill.

- Top whole wheat pizzettas with grilled vegetables instead of high-sodium and high-fat toppings such as pepperoni and Italian sausage.
- Baste a medley of acorn squash, butternut squash, carrots, parsnips, rutabaga, or turnips with olive oil. Sprinkle with fresh grated nutmeg and ground black pepper, then roast until tender.
- Sauté broccoli, broccolini, red onion, garlic, green beans, shiitake or crimini mushrooms, red bell pepper, and canned or frozen water chestnuts in garlic, olive oil, and low-sodium soy sauce.
- Try spicy jalapeño, scotch bonnet, habanero, and serrano peppers in your chicken, lamb, and beef dishes.

Starchy Carbohydrates

If your diet consists of white potatoes, white rice, and pasta and bread made from refined flour, then you are like the majority of Americans. Small changes in your diet, however, will help you achieve optimal health and prevent your high blood pressure from rising further.

The much-maligned white potato is actually nutritious if not deep-fried or combined with heavy amounts of salt, butter, heavy cream, cheese, sour cream, and bacon bits. With the shortage of rice worldwide from recent natural disasters, white potatoes are now being planted by farmers to sustain many poorer countries. Roasted or baked sweet potatoes are great choices and are also great sources of vitamins.

Try these healthier approaches to eating potatoes:

- Peel and dice sweet potatoes, baste with a light coating of olive oil, orange zest, and cinnamon, then roast or bake covered with foil until tender.
- Boil washed and unpeeled red-skin potatoes and smash with olive oil, red cayenne pepper flakes, garlic, chives, and light sour cream.
- Roast washed and unpeeled red new potatoes with dried rosemary, garlic, and ground black or red cayenne pepper, and baste with olive oil. Bake until tender and browned.
- Wash and baste small three-inch potatoes with olive oil and bake until tender. Top with snipped chives and a tablespoon of light sour cream.

- Combine boiled red potatoes with chopped celery, red and green bell peppers, cayenne pepper flakes, sweet pickle, and a splash of vinegar to warm potatoes. Dress with an aioli of plain nonfat yogurt, Dijon mustard, light mayonnaise, and fresh snipped dill for a reduced-calorie summer potato salad.

Fill Up on Fiber

Don't forget about dietary fiber, the indigestible portion of plant foods that moves food through the digestive system. Fiber doesn't have its own food group per se, but maybe it should be the fifth food group for all the benefits provided, and it's a major component of the Mediterranean diet. In fact, when people ask me, "What is the most commonly deficient part of the American diet?" I say fiber. Most adults should eat at least 35 grams of fiber daily. Part of the problem is that many people don't even know where fiber resides or what it does.

Fiber cleanses the digestive system, keeps bowel movements regular, and may guard against cancer. Fiber is found in fruits, vegetables, beans, and whole grains.

Whole grains are critical in keeping blood pressure low, according to studies, my observation, and the *American Journal of Clinical Nutrition*. In the 2007 *Clinical Nutrition* study, women participants who ate at least one serving of whole grains saw their odds of developing high blood pressure over a decade fall by 4 percent. That may not sound like a whopping advantage. But since high blood pressure makes heart attacks, strokes, and a host of other health problems more likely, every little step helps.

Out of 29,000 survey participants, 8,722 women were newly diagnosed with high blood pressure. Women who reported eating at least four daily servings of whole grains were nearly 25 percent less likely to be diagnosed with high blood pressure than women who said they ate less than half a daily serving during the study. Other factors, including age, vigorous exercise, smoking, and other dietary habits did not affect these survey findings. This study, as well as the existing body of medical research, makes a strong case for a diet rich in whole grains.

Brown Rice, Whole Wheat Pasta, Quinoa, Bulgur Wheat, Couscous, and Barley

A large variety of pasta is now available in whole wheat varieties. Brown rice, whole-wheat pasta, whole-grain quinoa, whole-grain bulgur wheat, whole wheat couscous, and whole-grain barley can be combined with fresh produce, small amounts of chicken breast, and low-sodium chicken, beef, or fish stock to produce low-calorie, low-fat vegetable soups. One serving of rice and pasta is half a cup.

Try these combinations:

- Blanche bite-size pieces of fresh asparagus, broccoli, and green beans for one to two minutes. Chill in ice water to retain green color and stop cooking. Add chopped garlic, red onion, bell pepper, celery, and grilled chicken, salmon, or shrimp to cooked whole wheat bowtie pasta and dress with low-sodium vinaigrette dressing. Serve chilled as is or over salad greens.
- Grill shiitake mushrooms, zucchini, tomatoes, and red onion. Mince into smaller pieces and add minced garlic, fresh basil, and oregano to replace ground meat in lasagna recipes. Spread between layers of whole wheat lasagna noodles. Top with fire-roasted tomato sauce and reduced-fat mozzarella cheese.
- Cook brown rice with low-fat/low-sodium chicken stock, herbs, vegetables, and dried fruit to enhance flavor.
- Quinoa, bulgur wheat, and couscous are fast-swelling grains that require very little prep time and can be eaten hot as a side dish or cold combined with vegetables in salads. See recipe section for serving suggestions.

Whole-Grain Breads and Cereals

A variety of whole-grain breads and cereals are now available in most supermarkets, including whole wheat pita, flat breads, crackers, English muffins, and tortillas. Several recipes for whole-grain breads and breakfast breads are available in the recipe section. Both hot and cold dry cereals are recommended for light meals any time of day. Reading labels is important, since many manufacturers add salt and sugar to make them more palatable.

Whole-grain bread product tips:

- When choosing whole-grain products, look for products that list a whole grain first in the ingredient statement. Product names and information on product labels may be deceiving. For instance, a bread product labeled "wheat bread" will often list enriched wheat flour as the first ingredient.

- Whole wheat tortillas are an excellent choice for sandwich wraps.
- Breads containing significant whole grains are quite filling. You'll be less hungry after eating a hearty whole-grain slice for breakfast with a small amount of jam and natural peanut butter.
- Baked goods do contain salt for flavor and leavening. In moderation, they can be included in a diet for bringing down high blood pressure.
- Old-fashioned oats cook in five minutes for a quick breakfast. The oats can also be added dry to meat loaf, meatball, and hamburger recipes to keep lean ground meat from becoming too dry during the cooking process.
- Try cereals with significant amounts of whole grain. Remember to look for a whole grain listed first in the ingredient statement before selecting a cereal product.

Fresh Fruit, Fruit Juice, Frozen Fruit, and Dried Fruit

You can't go wrong with fruit: oranges, tangerines, apples, oranges, pears, peaches, nectarines, clementines, grapefruit, grapes, tangelos, cherries, watermelon, bananas, cantaloupe, and pineapple. Fresh fruit is rich in key antioxidant vitamins as well as macronutrients such as potassium. Fresh whole fruit is preferable, but fruit juice is a readily accessible way of increasing your fruit consumption.

Don't rush to embrace fruit juice, however. Fruit juice is metabolized more rapidly and may cause blood sugar spikes if you are diabetic. If you are diabetic, you should consume fruit juice in moderation.

When you select juices, look for 100 percent unsweetened juice—fruit offers enough sugar on its own. Some juices also offer additional nutrients, such as calcium-fortified orange juice. Also, the FDA has approved a health claim related to heart disease risk reduction for Minute Maid® Heart Wise™ Orange Juice. This product contains plant sterol esters, which have been shown to have cholesterol-lowering effects.

Frozen Fruit

Unsweetened peaches, mangoes, strawberries, raspberries, blueberries, and cherries can now be found in the frozen food section and are useful for adding to recipes during off-seasons when fresh fruits are not available.

Dried Fruit

Dates, plums (prunes), cranberries, blueberries, figs, apricots, pears, peaches, apples, and raisins are excellent snacks to satisfy cravings for sweetness. Asian fruits such as dragonfruit and rambutan are available in dried varieties at specialty food stores. However, it is important that people with diabetes realize dried fruit is relatively high in sugar. Dried apricots are wonderful additions to salads and hot fruit compotes. They are naturally low in sodium and rich in fiber and nutrients, but dried fruit does contain calories and should be eaten in moderation.

Concerning Carbs

A question I often get in the health seminars I give is "What is the truth about carbohydrates?" There is some evidence that high-carbohydrate diets may actually increase blood pressure (especially in persons with diabetes), but this has not necessarily been substantiated.

The hype surrounding the low-carb craze certainly has a basis. However, you're likely not getting the full picture from your magazines or evening news shows. There are a variety of "low-carb" diets that are recommended for different reasons. Most of these regimens, like the Atkins Diet, are generally for weight loss and not for long-term use. Eating all the bacon, sausage, and steak you want at every meal won't benefit you or lower your blood pressure in the long run.

I'm not completely against carbohydrates, however. It is important to distinguish which carbohydrates are on the healthier end of the carb spectrum. My recommendation is not to eliminate carbohydrates from the diet, but to eat the right ones—the unrefined carbs.

So-called refined carbohydrates are not good in excess. Refined carbohydrates include white bread, white rice, white pasta, most crackers, sweets, jams, and jellies. They increase blood sugar levels and provide fewer relative nutrients than unrefined counterparts, thus earning them the nickname "empty calories." By keeping empty calories from your diet as much as possible (sometimes they sneak in), you can boost your nutrients and control your blood sugar and insulin levels. This is crucial if you have any form of diabetes, but especially type 2, and is also very important for weight maintenance even if you're diabetes-free.

Unrefined carbohydrates are kind to your body. Go ahead and eat carbohydrates in fruits, vegetables, and whole grains (i.e., brown rice, whole-grain cereals, stone ground whole-grain bread, whole wheat pasta, etc.). As we've seen in the sections on grains, there are many benefits such as energy and fiber found naturally in many of these products, and they are often enriched with vitamins and minerals as well. A high-carb diet isn't necessarily evil any more than a high-protein diet is.

Animal and Plant Proteins

Get your protein! Research indicates that protein-rich foods such as fish, chicken, dairy low in "bad fat," and lean meats can increase satiety, meaning they help you feel full longer. Think about it—do you eat more after you finish three dinner rolls (nonprotein) or three chicken breasts (protein)? If the dinner rolls are whole grain or baked without trans fats, fine, but if they're made with hydrogenated oils, they make you want to eat more and feel less satisfied, so that you do eat more.

Eat protein with every meal, and you'll curb your enthusiasm for snacking. For example, eggs, which have gained a bad rap, are one of the most affordable and delicious forms of protein and are actually low in fat. The protein is mainly found in the egg white. Limit the yolks due to high LDL cholesterol (the bad variety) content. Also, one half cup of beans contains as much protein as three ounces of steak (good news for vegetarians). Pork, the most widely eaten meat, is exceptionally lean (although slightly higher in fat than skinless chicken).

We hear many conflicting studies that suggest animal protein and meat are bad for you. If you're reluctant to give up chicken, beef, fish, pork, or eggs, take heart: Animal proteins don't automatically damage your heart and blood pressure if you consume them in moderation as part of a diet that includes plant proteins as well. Blood pressure-friendly fish and animal proteins include:

- White meat chicken or turkey (remove skin).
- Fish and shellfish (grilled, broiled, or baked, not fried with batter).
- Beef: round, sirloin, tenderloin, and lean ground beef.
- Pork tenderloin.
- Farm-raised tilapia, catfish, and salmon are economical fish options along with canned and foil-packed tuna and salmon.
- On the other hand, if you are vegetarian or vegan, look for tempeh, tofu, and Boca brand meat substitutes, which contain soy protein (soy may help lower blood pressure and cholesterol

in women with high blood pressure and postmenopausal women with normal blood pressure).

- Also, if you are vegetarian, try dried beans and peas: lentils, pinto, black and kidney beans, black-eyed peas, chickpeas, and green peas.

The most important thing to remember is that proteinaceous foods (yes, that is a word) often have added salt. In addition, eating too much protein may increase urinary calcium loss, which may increase the risk of osteoporosis. A very-high-protein diet is especially risky for patients with diabetes because it can speed the progression, even for short lengths of time, of diabetic kidney disease, which ultimately affects blood pressure.

Not all forms of protein are good. There is also another type of protein related to heart disease and high blood pressure specifically: C-reactive protein (CRP). This inflammatory protein is actually manufactured by the body and is detrimental to heart health. Scientists have come to believe that high levels of inflammatory proteins in the bloodstream raise the risk of a heart attack. Now a study suggests they also contribute to high blood pressure. Researchers have found that individuals with high circulating levels of CRP in their blood are much more likely to develop high blood pressure in the future.

Fats and Oils

Fats often have the same type of effect on satiety (feeling full) as proteins, and can therefore have a positive effect on regulating calorie intake. That said, however, you need to be cautious with consumption of fats. Eating the right proteins translates into not eating excess "bad fats"—that is, no high-fat pork such as processed bacon, no (or limited) red meat. It is important to realize the distinction between unsaturated and saturated fat. Saturated fat is processed bacon, unsaturated fat is olive oil. By now everyone is aware of trans fats and the campaign to eliminate them. Table 3.4 provides sources of saturated fat.

When you do add fat to meals, such as using oil when cooking, it is important to understand which fats you can eat. Trans fats from partially hydrogenated oils should make up less than 1 percent of your daily calories. Trans fats, typically found in commercially baked goods and snacks as well as margarine, raise LDL (bad cholesterol) but also lower HDL (good cholesterol) and increase inflammation in the body.

Table 3.4. Saturated Fat Contents

Food	Saturated Fat (gr)
Cheddar cheese (processed), 1 slice	6
Butter, 1 tablespoon	7
Croissant, medium	7
Cheesecake, 1 serving	8
Ground beef, 100 percent lean 5-ounce patty	10
Premium chocolate ice cream, ½ cup	11
Italian sausage, 2 links	14
Porterhouse steak, 9 ounces	18

With the "Keeping It Simple" approach that I like to stick with, you should always eat olive oil, macadamia nut oil, and canola oil, and you will be fine with no questions asked. It becomes more complicated when people "mix and match" the healthy with unhealthy selections. For example, eating a greasy burger and fries cooked in trans fats, eating an apple and some peanut butter afterward, and justifying this as eating healthily misses the mark. You can't counteract an unhealthy selection with a healthy one.

It's tough to be consistent, especially when eating out in restaurants and on airplanes. Many restaurants do offer a variety of healthy options, but this is not always the case. Foods cooked in peanut oil and some other vegetable oils are good choices when options are limited. Ask your waiter for details about the special of the day. If the fat in which your food is prepared is liquid at room temperature, it's a good bet that, in doctor-speak, a "large percentage of the chains on the triglyceride molecules" are unsaturated. In other words, these fats are often referred to as "oils" and are most likely better for your heart health. The vast majority of your fat calories should come from unsaturated fats, the kind found in most fish, nuts, seeds, and vegetable oils.

Substituting butter, lard, and other saturated fats with olive oil, canola, flaxseed, and soybean oils promotes heart health. Look for extra virgin olive oil with a "use-by" date as far into the future as possible. Don't purchase olive oil without an expiration date. Unlike fine wines, olive oil does not improve with age and can become rancid with exposure to high room temperature, light, and air.

Scientific studies have demonstrated the advantage of using virgin olive oil over refined olive oil since virgin olive oil tends to raise the good HDL cholesterol better than refined olive oil. Replacing saturated fats with extra virgin olive oil will help decrease total serum cholesterol and LDL cholesterol. Canola oil is a less pricey alternative to olive oil.

Butter is rich in fat, but margarine—which as I mentioned is high in trans fats—can be just as bad. If you eliminate butter and margarine altogether, look for alternatives such as low-cholesterol spread containing omega-3s.

Nuts

Try unsalted toasted almonds, peanuts, walnuts, cashews, and pecans.

- Many supermarkets and specialty health food stores now stock sodium-free and lightly salted nuts.
- Look for natural peanut or almond butter without trans fat or sugar.

Herbs and Spices

The use of herbs and spices to create full-bodied flavors instead of salt may take some adjusting to, but the avoidance of salt and salty foods and snacks is crucial to managing high blood pressure. Chapter 4 provides a cornucopia of herbs, spices, and marinades to make you forget your salt craving. And of course I would be delighted for you to try my FlavorDoctor brand of seasoning. You can trust that its great flavor will also be low in sodium.

Dairy Products

Calcium, which is most often found in dairy products, has not been consistently shown to prevent high blood pressure, but is important for overall good health. Good sources of calcium are low-fat dairy foods and nonfat dairy products. If you are lactose intolerant or don't eat dairy, other foods are high in calcium, such as nondairy milk, yogurt, and cheese.

Although you are probably familiar with the different types of dairy and their nutritional value, there are so many options that everyone

Table 3.5. Dairy and Nondairy Sources of Calcium

Food	Serving Size	Calcium (mg)
Broccoli, raw	1 cup	42
Cheese, cheddar	1 ounce	204
Milk, fat-free or skim	1 cup	301
Perch	3 ounces	116
Salmon	3 ounces	181
Sardine	3 ounces	325
Spinach, cooked	1 cup	245
Turnip greens, cooked	1 cup	197
Tofu, soft	1 piece	133
Yogurt, plain, skim milk	8-ounce container	452

Values were obtained from the USDA Nutrient Database for Standard References, Release 15 for Calcium, Ca (mg) content of selected foods per common measure.

http://www.nal.usda.gov/fnic/foodcomp/Data/SR15/wtrank/wt_rank.html

needs a guide when shopping the dairy aisle at the grocery store. My top tips and suggestions for enjoying dairy, guilt-free:

- Look for fat-free or low-fat milk, yogurt, cheese, light sour cream, and cottage cheese. Fat-free or skim milk is an excellent source of calcium, vitamins, and protein without artery-clogging fat and cholesterol.
- Look for soybean-based margarine products without trans fat.
- As an alternative to cow's milk, try vanilla, chocolate, or plain soy milks.

Canned or Bottled Food

While nothing can surpass the splendor of summer tomatoes for marinara sauce, organic canned tomatoes and tomato sauce can be substituted during winter or off-season when superior-quality fresh tomatoes are not available. Look for low-sodium varieties. Other useful canned or bottled food items are sardines, salmon, water-packed albacore tuna, light fruit juices, no-sugar-added applesauce, and spiced or plain beets.

Soups

Homemade soups are filling and satisfying. Soups made with beans or lentils and other vegetables are not only healthy but provide a satisfying meal. They are inexpensive, convenient, and easy to prepare. Low-sodium canned soups can serve as a snack, part of a meal, or as a base for adding fresh vegetables to prepare a full-bodied soup with brown rice, barley, and other whole grains. Organic brands as well as the canned soup varieties you grew up with now offer low-sodium and low-fat options.

Beverages

Plain tap water should be your first choice. Despite sales of over 17 billion dollars in 2007, bottled waters don't offer any benefit above city water as long as there are no water quality issues in your city. Use bottled water if your city water doesn't taste good or you suspect contamination.

- Drink at least 64 ounces of water per day (or eight glasses).
- Try unsweetened black coffee and tea as well as noncaffeinated herb tea such as green tea and Red Zinger tea.
- Consider flavored zero-calorie carbonated waters: orange, cranberry, lemon-lime, or maybe seltzer, club soda, Pellegrino, and Perrier sparkling water. These zero-calorie mixers are good mixed with equal parts purple grape, pomegranate, orange, and other natural, no-sugar-added fruit juice and wines.
- A glass of red wine is healthy and allowed in moderation.

Note: If you've been drinking more than one (for women) to two (for men) drinks a day, you'll have to cut back to protect your liver from further harm.

The Beverage Guidance Panel at the University of North Carolina grouped beverages into six categories, ranked them from most important to least important, and provided recommended daily amounts of each to meet the requirements. Here are their suggestions:

- Level 1 (most important)—Water: 20 to 50 fl. ounces/day
- Level 2: Tea and coffee—0 to 40 fluid ounces/day (can replace an equivalent amount of water); limit caffeine intake to no more than 400 milligrams/day

- Level 3: Low-fat/skim milk and soy beverages—0 to 16 fluid ounces/day
- Level 4: Noncaloric sweetened beverages (e.g., Diet Coke®)—0 to 32 fluid ounces/day
- Level 5: Caloric beverages with some nutrients (e.g., 100 percent fruit juices, alcohol)—Fruit juices: 0 to 8 fluid ounces/day; Alcohol: 0 to 1 drinks per day for women, 0 to 2 drinks per day for men.
- Level 6 (least important)—Caloric sweetened beverages (e.g., nondiet soft drinks): 0 to 8 fluid ounces/day

Caffeine in coffee, tea, chocolate, cocoa, and soft drinks can affect blood pressure. Fortunately, in liquid form, caffeine only raises blood pressure temporarily, especially in people who don't consume caffeine regularly. Most people with high blood pressure should be able to enjoy coffee, tea, and other caffeine-containing beverages and food in moderation.

If you are sensitive to caffeine and notice a spike in your blood pressure after caffeine consumption, then restrict your diet to avoid caffeine. For many people, the amount of caffeine in two to three cups of coffee has been shown to raise blood pressure significantly. Some researchers suggest caffeine narrows blood vessels by blocking the effects of adenosine, a hormone that helps keep them widened. Caffeine may also stimulate the adrenal glands to release more cortisol and adrenaline, which is known to increase blood pressure.

At the very least, caffeine consumption should be controlled. Many experts suggest a maximum of 200 milligrams a day, or two twelve-ounce cups of brewed coffee. But even this amount may be too high for caffeine-sensitive people with elevated blood pressure.

To see if caffeine might be raising your blood pressure, check your blood pressure within 30 minutes of drinking a cup of coffee or another caffeinated beverage you regularly consume. If your blood pressure increases by five to ten points, you may be sensitive to the blood-pressure-raising effects of caffeine. If you plan to reduce your intake of caffeine, do so gradually over several days to a week to avoid withdrawal headaches.

Nutrition Is More Than What You Eat or Drink

By now you might have highlighted and marked up this entire section. You may also be overwhelmed with all the smart shopping suggestions, even if you've heard them before. Your brain is stuffed with lists of items to remember. You may even be panicking.

People who attend my seminars often express frustration with diet. The complaints I hear most often are:

- "Whole wheat, whole-grain, fat-free, I have difficulty keeping track of it all."
- "I feel guilty if I'm not eating enough fruits and vegetables, which I'm usually not. But who has time to eat right?"
- "Forget diet. It's all about the supplements you take, isn't it?"
- "It's all about exercise, you just said. It doesn't matter what I eat."

Let me answer some of these assertions and clear up any misconceptions as best I can.

With regard to exercise, I've talked about it in the previous chapter and will discuss it in detail in Chapter 6. I always believe that exercise and diet, like love and marriage, go hand in hand. You can't practice healthy eating without exercise. Your calorie intake and your level of physical activity are directly related. Also, you can be the most athletic person in the world, but if you're not getting the right nutrients, your health and your blood pressure will suffer eventually, as scientific evidence shows. I stand by what I write in this book, including the need to take the time to invest in your own health.

I agree that it's often inconvenient to think about what you're eating or what you should be eating. Some of the patients at our health facility find it helpful to keep a food diary. A gifted nutritionist such as my collaborator on this book, Sarah Schein, can write out a detailed plan. A nutritionist can include any necessary vitamin or mineral supplements.

People often tell me that they don't have time to eat right. I admit it is easier to just microwave a frozen pizza or breeze through the drive-through. It's easier to take the attitude of the young mother I mentioned in the last chapter. Our lives are overwhelming and over-stuffed. Our stress levels have risen to epic proportions, especially with the economic crisis.

However, I believe that eating right and taking the time for nutrition ease our stress and create more time in our lives. Consider the amount of money that people spend on fast food and the "latte factor," getting a latte (or doughnut) every morning on your way to work. A burst of caffeine, sugar, salt, and fat, and you feel unsatisfied and irritable later. You begin to crave more fast food instead of the healthy, delicious food that is yours for the asking. You spend more time ill and tired and always hungry for the food you have trained yourself to want.

Here are some time-saving tips to help you eat the way your body intended.

- Buy fresh fruits and vegetables that are ripe or near-ripe, and place them in your refrigerator or on your counter in immediate reach whenever you're hungry.
- Pack sandwich bags full of nuts or dried fruit for easy snacking during the day.
- Invest in a juicer for fruits and vegetables. A no-frills basic juicer can cost under $100 at Target. You can't beat fresh fruit or vegetable juice! You can even splurge on juicers online that will last years with low-price guarantees. The Internet makes it easy to shop for juicers. In addition, you can use juicers to create delicious salsas and vegetable or fruit purees.
- Invest in a fruit and vegetable dehydrator if you want to keep produce from spoiling while preserving essential nutrients and taste. Your cost of dehydrating food averages pennies a day, and dehydrated produce is easy to store.
- Buy an indoor herb container garden and grow your own herbs. This is a terrific project for children or the gardener in the household.
- Buy bulk lean turkey, beef, or chicken at Costco or Sam's Club.
- Keep a list of meals you can make ahead of time or that take 30 minutes or less to prepare. Be sure to mark which ones are family favorites. Keep it on the refrigerator or in another spot where you can look at it every day.

- Keep a tally of the money and time you've saved while you chart your blood pressure readings—you'll become motivated to continue eating right!
- If cooking has become a chore or if you hate to cook, find a way to make it enjoyable. Give recipe suggestions to someone who enjoys cooking and plan meals together. You can do the shopping while your friend does the cooking. Think outside the takeout box.

Cooking Creatively

Exploring different flavors and textures can open up an entire new cooking world. For instance, subscribing to a health-oriented cooking magazine can provide creative new ideas to bring into your traditional menus. You can aim to try new recipes that combine different colors.

Colorful is good! Experts have suggested that the typical American diet consists of dull colors like brown and tan—is your diet close to this spectrum? Creatively introduce bright colors from fruits and vegetables into your menus. Radiant-hued items typically provide many beneficial vitamins, minerals, and phytonutrients. The bottom line is that these can help protect our bodies from chronic diseases and augment overall health.

The recipes in the next section are certainly creative and dynamic. Adding them to your repertoire will help you in your mission. The recipes have been chosen according to nutrition, blood-pressure-lowering effects, ease of preparation, and taste. Try some of these recipes, which certainly shouldn't bore even the toughest connoisseurs.

Chapter 4

DELICIOUS RECIPES FOR BRINGING DOWN HIGH BLOOD PRESSURE

NOTE THAT SOME of these recipes call for egg substitute wherever possible to reduce cholesterol. However, these recipes have been kitchen-tested and they taste great! Cooking oil spray is also used to cut back on fat.

Many of these recipes are delicious with my FlavorDoctor seasoning, an excellent way to simplify cooking. When you see an asterisk (*) next to a spice or flavoring in the recipes, substitute one or more shakes—to your taste—of FlavorDoctor for that spice.

To find out more information and to order FlavorDoctor, visit http://www.shop.youroptimumhealth.net.

APPETIZERS

Pupusas Revueltas with Chicken

YIELD: 12 SERVINGS

Ingredients

1 pound ground chicken
1 tbsp vegetable oil
½ small onion, finely diced
1 garlic clove, minced*
1 medium green pepper, seeded and minced
1 small tomato, finely chopped
½ tsp salt
5 cups instant corn flour (masa harina)
6 cups water
½ pound low-fat mozzarella cheese, grated

1. In a nonstick skillet over low heat, sauté chicken in oil until chicken turns white. Constantly stir the chicken to keep it from sticking.

2. Add onion, garlic, green pepper, and tomato. Cook until chicken mixture is cooked through. Remove skillet from stove and let mixture cool in the refrigerator.

3. While the chicken mixture is cooling, place the flour in a large mixing bowl and stir in enough water to make a stiff, tortilla-like dough.

4. When the chicken mixture has cooled, mix in the cheese.

5. Divide the dough into 24 portions. With your hands, roll the dough into balls and flatten each ball into a ½-inch-thick circle. Put a

spoonful of the chicken mixture in the middle of each circle of dough and bring the edges to the center. Flatten the ball of dough again until it is ½ inch thick.

6. In a very hot iron skillet, cook the pupusas on each side until golden brown.

NUTRITION

Serving size: 2 pupusas
Each serving provides:
Calories: 291
Total fat: 6.5 g
    Saturated fat: 3 g
    Monounsaturated fat: 2 g
    Polyunsaturated fat: 1.5 g
Cholesterol: 31 mg
Sodium: 211 mg
Potassium: 339 mg

Carbohydrates: 41 g
Sugar: 7 g
Total fiber: 4 g
Protein: 17 g
Iron: 2 mg
Magnesium: 79 mg
Calcium: 149 mg
Vitamin A: 0 IU
Vitamin C: 8 mg
Vitamin D: 0 µg

Spicy and Sweet Meatballs

Ingredients

¼ cup onion, chopped

1 pound lean ground beef

⅓ cup fine dried breadcrumbs

¼ cup fresh parsley, chopped

⅛ tsp nutmeg*

¼ cup liquid nondairy creamer

1 egg white, beaten

½ cup cranberries, finely chopped

2 tsp dry mustard*

⅛ tsp cayenne pepper*

½ cup grape jelly

1 tsp lemon juice

1. Coat small saucepan with cooking spray; place over medium heat.
2. Add onion and sauté until tender.
3. Combine onion with next six ingredients in a bowl. Shape into thirty-six 1-inch meatballs. Place meatballs on a cooking spray–coated baking sheet (with sides) and bake at 375°F for 18 minutes.
4. Meanwhile, prepare sauce by combining the cranberries and remaining ingredients in a small saucepan. Cook over medium heat until thoroughly heated.
5. Place meatballs in a serving bowl and pour the sauce over. Serve with toothpicks.

NUTRITION	
Serving size: 3 meatballs	Carbohydrates: 12 g
Each serving provides:	Sugar: 2 g
Calories: 95	Total fiber: 0.5 g
Total fat: 1.2 g	Protein: 9 g
Saturated fat: 0.5 g	Iron: 1 mg
Monounsaturated fat: 0.7 g	Magnesium: 11 mg
Polyunsaturated fat: 0 g	Calcium: 12 mg
Cholesterol: 20 mg	Vitamin A: 7 IU
Sodium: 55 mg	Vitamin C: 2 mg
Potassium: 156 mg	Vitamin D: 0 µg

Curtido Cabbage Salvadore

YIELD: 8 SERVINGS

Ingredients

1 medium head cabbage, chopped

2 small carrots, grated

1 small onion, sliced

½ tsp dried red pepper (optional)

½ tsp oregano*

1 tsp olive oil

1 tsp light salt

1 tsp brown sugar

¼ cup vinegar

½ cup water

1. Blanch the cabbage with boiling water for 1 minute. Discard the water.
2. Place the cabbage in a large bowl and add grated carrots, sliced onion, red pepper, oregano, olive oil, salt, brown sugar, vinegar, and water.
3. Place in refrigerator for at least 2 hours before serving.
4. Serve with Pupusas Revueltas (page 56).

NUTRITION	
Serving size: 1 cup	Carbohydrates: 6 g
Each serving provides:	Sugar: <1 g
Calories: 37	Total fiber: 1.5 g
Total fat: 1 g	Protein: 1 g
Saturated fat: 0 g	Iron: 0.5 mg
Monounsaturated fat: 0.5 g	Magnesium: 10 mg
Polyunsaturated fat: 0.5 g	Calcium: 27 mg
Cholesterol: 0 mg	Vitamin A: 516 IU
Sodium: 293 mg	Vitamin C: 14 mg
Potassium: 375 mg	Vitamin D: 0 µg

Mexican Pozole

Ingredients

1 tbsp olive oil

2 pounds lean beef, cubed (see note)

1 large onion, chopped

1 clove garlic, finely chopped*

¼ tsp light salt

⅛ tsp black pepper*

¼ cup cilantro*

1 can (15 oz) stewed tomatoes

2 oz tomato paste (no added salt)

1 can (1 lb, 13 oz) hominy

Note: Skinless, boneless chicken can be used instead of beef cubes.

1. In large pot, heat oil, then sauté beef.
2. Add onion, garlic, salt, pepper, cilantro, and enough water to cover meat. Cover pot and cook over low heat until meat is tender.
3. Add tomatoes and tomato paste. Continue cooking for about 20 minutes.
4. Add hominy and continue cooking over low heat for another 15 minutes, stirring occasionally. If too thick, add water for desired consistency.

NUTRITION	
Each serving provides:	Carbohydrates: 18 g
Calories: 214	Sugar: 4 g
Total fat: 6 g	Total fiber: 2 g
Saturated fat: 3 g	Protein: 22 g
Monounsaturated fat: 2.5 g	Iron: 6.5 mg
Polyunsaturated fat: 0.5 g	Magnesium: 30 mg
Cholesterol: 48 mg	Calcium: 29 mg
Sodium: 328 mg	Vitamin A: 25 IU
Potassium: 420 mg	Vitamin C: 4 mg
	Vitamin D: 0.2 µg

Spicy Marinated Shrimp Bowl

Ingredients

5 pounds fresh large shrimp, peeled and deveined

½ cup olive oil

½ cup white or red vinegar

1½ tsp lemon peel, finely shredded

¼ cup lemon juice

2 tbsp tomato paste (no added salt)

3 garlic cloves, minced*

½ tsp light salt

¼ tsp cayenne pepper*

1 tsp black pepper*

½ tsp white pepper, ground*

1. In a large kettle, bring 5 quarts water to a boil and then add shrimp. Bring to a boil again, and then reduce heat to a simmer. Simmer, uncovered, for 1 to 3 minutes or until shrimp is done. Drain shrimp. Rinse under cold running water; drain again.

2. For marinade, in a screw-top jar combine oil, vinegar, lemon peel, lemon juice, tomato paste, garlic, salt, and all 3 types of pepper. Cover and shake well. Pour marinade over shrimp. Cover and chill overnight.

NUTRITION

Each serving provides:	
Calories: 207	Carbohydrates: 2.5 g
Total fat: 8.5 g	Sugar: 0 g
Saturated fat: 1.5 g	Total fiber: 0 g
Monounsaturated fat: 5.5 g	Protein: 30 g
Polyunsaturated fat: 1.5 g	Iron: 3.8 mg
Cholesterol: 229 mg	Magnesium: 58 mg
Sodium: 265 mg	Calcium: 82 mg
Potassium: 369 mg	Vitamin A: 88 IU
	Vitamin C: 6 mg
	Vitamin D: 5.5 µg

Black-Eyed Pea Salsa

YIELD: 4 SERVINGS

Ingredients

1 can (15 oz) black-eyed peas, rinsed and drained
¼ cup thinly sliced green onion
¼ cup red sweet pepper, chopped
2 tbsp canola oil
2 tbsp cider vinegar
1 to 2 fresh jalapeño peppers, seeded and chopped
¼ tsp black pepper*
2 cloves garlic, minced*

1. In a bowl, combine all ingredients, cover, and chill overnight.

NUTRITION

Serving size: ½ cup
Each serving provides:
Calories: 169
Total fat: 6.5 g
  Saturated fat: 0.5 g
  Monounsaturated fat: 4 g
  Polyunsaturated fat: 2 g
Cholesterol: 0 mg
Sodium: 147 mg
Potassium: 507 mg

Carbohydrates: 24 g
  Sugar: 0 g
  Total fiber: 5 g
Protein: 3.5 g
Iron: 1.6 mg
Magnesium: 61 mg
Calcium: 146 mg
Vitamin A: 135 IU
Vitamin C: 22 mg
Vitamin D: 0 µg

Pan-Fried Yucca

Ingredients

1 pound fresh yucca (cassava, cut into 3-inch sections and peeled)

1. In a kettle, combine the yucca with enough cold water to cover it by 1 inch. Bring the water to a boil, and slowly simmer the yucca for 20 to 30 minutes, or until it is tender.
2. Preheat oven to 350°F.
3. Transfer the yucca with a slotted spoon to a cutting board, let it cool, and cut it lengthwise into ¾-inch-wide wedges, discarding the thin woody core.
4. Spray cookie sheet with cooking spray. Spread yucca wedges on cookie sheet, and spray wedges with cooking spray. Cover with foil paper and bake for 8 minutes. Uncover and return to oven to bake for an additional 7 minutes.

NUTRITION

Serving size: 1 piece	Carbohydrates: 28 g
(2½ inches long)	Sugar: 5 g
Each serving provides:	Total fiber: 1 g
Calories: 116	Protein: 1 g
Total fat: <1 g	Iron: 3 mg
Saturated fat: <1 g	Magnesium: 15 mg
Monounsaturated fat: 0 g	Calcium: 66 mg
Polyunsaturated fat: 0 g	Vitamin A: 1.5 IU
Cholesterol: 0 mg	Vitamin C: 15.5 mg
Sodium: 3 mg	Vitamin D: 0 µg
Potassium: 205 mg	

Roasted Red Pepper Hummus

Ingredients

1 can (16 oz) chickpeas or garbanzo beans

1½ tsp cumin*

1 tsp coriander

¼ tsp cayenne pepper*

½ tsp light salt

2 tbsp tahini

1 tbsp lemon juice

2 to 3 cloves garlic, pressed or crushed*

½ cup roasted red pepper

Fresh ground pepper to taste*

1. Drain and rinse chickpeas/garbanzos, reserving liquid.
2. In small bowl, combine cumin, coriander, cayenne, and salt. Mix thoroughly.
3. Put chickpeas in bowl of food processor with chopping blade and sprinkle the spice mixture over the top evenly.
4. Add the tahini, lemon juice, garlic, and roasted red pepper, and blend until well mixed. Add the fresh ground pepper to taste.
5. Once the hummus is smooth, add some of the reserved liquid from the chickpeas while it is being processed, until it reaches the desired consistency.
6. Serve with toasted pita bread or as a dip or spread with almost anything.

NUTRITION	
Each serving provides:	Carbohydrates: 23 g
Calories: 156	Sugar: 4 g
Total fat: 4 g	Total fiber: 6 g
Saturated fat: 0.5 g	Protein: 7 g
Monounsaturated fat: 1.5 g	Iron: 2.5 mg
Polyunsaturated fat: 2 g	Magnesium: 55 mg
Cholesterol: 0 mg	Calcium: 47 mg
Sodium: 103 mg	Vitamin A: 41 IU
Potassium: 394 mg	Vitamin C: 14 mg
	Vitamin D: 0 µg

Gazpacho

Ingredients

3 medium tomatoes, peeled and chopped

½ cup cucumber, seeded and chopped

½ cup green pepper, chopped

2 green onions, sliced

2 cups low-sodium vegetable juice cocktail

1 tbsp lemon juice

½ tsp basil, dried*

¼ tsp hot pepper sauce*

1 clove garlic, minced*

1. In large mixing bowl, combine all ingredients.
2. Cover and chill in the refrigerator for several hours.

NUTRITION

Each serving provides:	
Calories: 65	Carbohydrates: 12 g
Total fat: 1 g	Sugar: 1 g
Saturated fat: 0.5 g	Total fiber: 2 g
Monounsaturated fat: 0 g	Protein: 2 g
Polyunsaturated fat: 0.5 g	Iron: 1 mg
Cholesterol: 0 mg	Magnesium: 15 mg
Sodium: 41 mg	Calcium: 47 mg
Potassium: 514 mg	Vitamin A: 178 IU
	Vitamin C: 62 mg
	Vitamin D: 0 µg

Pesto Pita Bites

Ingredients

1 cup fresh basil leaves, packed*

2 garlic cloves, finely minced*

2 to 3 tbsp Parmesan cheese

¼ cup olive oil

1 whole pita bread

1. Place basil leaves in a food processor until well chopped. Add the garlic and 1½ tablespoons of the Parmesan cheese and blend while slowly adding the olive oil.
2. Split pita bread into 2 rounds. Spread with pesto mix and sprinkle with cheese.
3. Cut each into 6 wedges and then place on an ungreased baking sheet.
4. Bake at 350°F for 10 to 12 minutes or until crisp. Serve warm.

NUTRITION

Each serving provides:	
Calories: 228	Carbohydrates: 20 g
Total fat: 14 g	Sugar: 6 g
Saturated fat: 2.5 g	Total fiber: 8.5 g
Monounsaturated fat: 10 g	Protein: 5.5 g
Polyunsaturated fat: 1.5 g	Iron: 9 mg
Cholesterol: 2.5 mg	Magnesium: 89 mg
Sodium: 150 mg	Calcium: 428 mg
Potassium: 654 mg	Vitamin A: 174 IU
	Vitamin C: 11.5 mg
	Vitamin D: 0 µg

BREADS

Hawaiian Bread

YIELD: 12 SERVINGS PER LOAF

Ingredients

⅓ cup sugar

⅓ cup margarine

½ cup egg substitute

2 cups flour

3 tsp baking powder

1 cup crushed pineapple (in its own juice), drained

6 maraschino cherries, chopped

1. Beat sugar and margarine until light and fluffy.
2. Add egg substitute and mix well.
3. Mix flour and baking powder together in a separate bowl. Combine sugar and flour mixtures. Blend.
4. Add pineapple and cherries and mix to combine. Pour into greased 9- × 5-inch pan.
5. Bake at 350°F for 1 hour.

NUTRITION

Each serving provides:	
Calories: 136	Carbohydrates: 26 g
Total fat: 2 g	Sugar: 10 g
Saturated fat: 0.5 g	Total fiber: 1 g
Monounsaturated fat: 0.5 g	Protein: 3.5 g
Polyunsaturated fat: 1 g	Iron: 1.2 mg
Cholesterol: <1 mg	Magnesium: 8.5 mg
Sodium: 51 mg	Calcium: 12 mg
Potassium: 87 mg	Vitamin A: 47.8 IU
	Vitamin C: 2 mg
	Vitamin D: <1 μg

Raspberry Streusel Muffins

YIELD: 16 MUFFINS

Ingredients

1⅓ cups flour
1½ tsp baking powder
1 cup fresh or frozen raspberries
¼ cup margarine
½ cup sugar
¼ cup egg substitute
½ cup liquid nondairy creamer
¼ cup brown sugar
¼ cup flour
2 tbsp margarine
2 tsp cinnamon

1. Preheat oven to 375°F. Line 16 muffin cups with paper liners.
2. Mix 1⅓ cups flour and baking powder in a small bowl. Stir in raspberries.
3. In a separate bowl, beat ¼ cup margarine with sugar and egg substitute. Blend in creamer.
4. Stir in flour mixture until just moistened. Spoon into 16 muffin cups.
5. In a small bowl, mix brown sugar, ¼ cup flour, 2 tbsp margarine, and cinnamon. Sprinkle over muffins and bake for approximately 15 minutes.

NUTRITION

Serving size: 1 muffin	Carbohydrates: 23 g
Each serving provides:	Sugar: 6 g
Calories: 118	Total fiber: 1 g
Total fat: 2 g	Protein: 1.8 g
Saturated fat: 0.5 g	Iron: 1 mg
Monounsaturated fat: 0.5 g	Magnesium: 5.5 mg
Polyunsaturated fat: 1 g	Calcium: 37 mg
Cholesterol: <1 mg	Vitamin A: 28.5 IU
Sodium: 81 mg	Vitamin C: 2 mg
Potassium: 53 mg	Vitamin D: <1 µg

Zucchini Bread

Ingredients

¾ cup egg substitute

1½ cups sugar

1 cup applesauce

2 cups unpeeled zucchini, shredded

1 tsp vanilla

2 cups flour

¼ tsp baking powder

1 tsp baking soda

1 tsp cinnamon

½ tsp ginger

1 cup unsalted chopped nuts

1. Beat egg substitute.
2. Mix sugar, applesauce, zucchini, and vanilla into eggs.
3. In a separate bowl, sift dry ingredients together and add to mixture.
4. Pour into a loaf pan and bake at 375°F for 1 hour.
5. Cut into 16 slices.

NUTRITION

Each serving provides:	
Calories: 200	Carbohydrates: 35 g
Total fat: 4.5 g	Sugar: 12 g
Saturated fat: 0.5 g	Total fiber: 1.5 g
Monounsaturated fat: 1 g	Protein: 5 g
Polyunsaturated fat: 3 g	Iron: 1.3 mg
Cholesterol: <1 mg	Magnesium: 21.5 mg
Sodium: 108 mg	Calcium: 20 mg
Potassium: 118 mg	Vitamin A: 29 IU
	Vitamin C: 1.4 mg
	Vitamin D: <1 µg

Whole Wheat Popovers

Ingredients

1¼ cups all-purpose flour

¾ cup whole wheat flour

¾ tsp salt

2 cups low-fat milk

1 cup egg substitute

2 tbsp melted butter, cooled

1. Preheat oven to 450°F.
2. In medium bowl, combine flours and salt.
3. In a separate bowl; with a blender at low speed, blend milk, egg substitute, and butter. Slowly add dry ingredients and process until smooth.
4. Spray two 12-cup muffin pans with cooking spray; pour in batter, filling each about ¾ full. Bake 15 minutes.
5. Reduce oven temperature to 350°F and bake an additional 15 to 20 minutes.

NUTRITION

Serving size: 2 popovers	Carbohydrates: 17 g
Each serving provides:	Sugar: 5 g
Calories: 107	Total fiber: 1.3 g
Total fat: 3 g	Protein: 3 g
Saturated fat: 1.5 g	Iron: 1 mg
Monounsaturated fat: 1 g	Magnesium: 20 mg
Polyunsaturated fat: 0.5 g	Calcium: 66 mg
Cholesterol: 7 mg	Vitamin A: 87 IU
Sodium: 151 mg	Vitamin C: 0.5 mg
Potassium: 275 mg	Vitamin D: 0.6 µg

Blueberry Oat Bran Muffins

Ingredients

1½ cups oat bran

1½ cups all-purpose flour

½ cup packed brown sugar

2 tsp baking soda

2 tsp baking powder

1 tsp ground cinnamon

½ tsp salt

1⅛ cups applesauce

½ cup egg substitute

2 tbsp canola oil

1 tsp vanilla extract

1½ cups blueberries

¼ ounce chopped pecans

½ cup low-fat granola

1. Preheat oven to 400°F. Line a 12-cup muffin pan with paper muffin liners, and spray liners with cooking spray.
2. In a large bowl, mix the oat bran, flour, brown sugar, baking soda, baking powder, cinnamon, and salt.
3. In a separate bowl, blend the applesauce, egg substitute, canola oil, and vanilla extract. Thoroughly mix the applesauce mixture into the flour mixture.
4. Fold in the blueberries and pecans. Spoon the batter into the prepared muffin cups. Sprinkle batter with granola, and press granola lightly to make it stick.
5. Bake 18 minutes in the preheated oven, or until a toothpick inserted into a muffin comes out clean. Cool on a wire rack.

NUTRITION

Serving size: 1 muffin

Each serving provides:

Calories: 218

Total fat: 4 g

  Saturated fat: 0.5 g

  Monounsaturated fat: 2 g

  Polyunsaturated fat: 1.5 g

Cholesterol: <1 mg

Sodium: 370 mg

Potassium: 260 mg

Carbohydrates: 40 g

Sugar: 15 g

Total fiber: 3.5 g

Protein: 5.5 g

Iron: 2 mg

Magnesium: 40 mg

Calcium: 72 mg

Vitamin A: 43 IU

Vitamin C: 2.8 mg

Vitamin D: <1 µg

Oatmeal Bread

Ingredients

4 cups all-purpose flour, plus additional for kneading
1 package active dry yeast
1¾ cups water
⅓ cup brown sugar
3 tbsp margarine
1 tsp salt
½ tsp cinnamon
2 cups rolled oats

1. In a large mixing bowl, combine 2 cups of all-purpose flour and yeast; set aside.
2. In medium saucepan, heat and stir water, brown sugar, margarine, salt, and cinnamon just until warm and the margarine almost melts. Add this liquid mixture to flour/yeast mixture.
3. Beat with an electric mixer on low to medium speed for 30 seconds. Then beat on high for 3 minutes. Then stir in rolled oats and the remaining all-purpose flour.
4. On a lightly floured surface, knead in enough of the all-purpose flour to make a moderately stiff dough that is smooth and elastic. Shape dough into a ball. Place dough in a lightly greased bowl; turn once to grease surface. Cover and let dough rise in a warm place until double in size (1 to 1½ hours).
5. Once dough has doubled in size, push your fist down into the center of the dough. Then turn out onto a lightly floured surface and divide in half.
6. Shape each dough half into a loaf by patting or rolling.
7. Place shaped dough halves into 2 lightly greased loaf pans. Cover and let rise in a warm place again until nearly double in size (~35 to 40 minutes).

8. Preheat oven to 375°F. Bake for 35 to 40 minutes. (May need to cover bread loosely with foil for the last 10 minutes to prevent overbrowning.) Immediately remove bread from loaf pans and cool on wire rack.

NUTRITION

Serving size: 12 servings per loaf

Each serving provides:

Calories: 103

Total fat: 1 g

    Saturated fat: <1 g

    Monounsaturated fat: <1 g

    Polyunsaturated fat: 0.5 g

Cholesterol: 0 mg

Sodium: 60 mg

Potassium: 115 mg

Carbohydrates: 21 g

    Sugar: 11 g

    Total fiber: 1 g

Protein: 2.5 g

Iron: 1 mg

Magnesium: 10.5 mg

Calcium: 8 mg

Vitamin A: 6.74 IU

Vitamin C: 0 mg

Vitamin D: 0 µg

English Muffin Bread

Ingredients

6 cups all-purpose flour

2 packages active dry yeast

¼ tsp baking soda

2 cups low-fat milk

½ cup water

1 tbsp sugar

1 tsp salt

¾ cup cornmeal

1. Grease 2 loaf pans and lightly sprinkle greased pans with cornmeal to coat bottoms and sides. Set pans aside.
2. In a large mixing bowl, combine ½ of the flour, yeast, and baking soda; set aside.
3. In a medium saucepan, heat and stir milk, water, sugar, and salt just until warm. Then stir milk mixture into flour mixture and stir in remaining flour.
4. Divide dough in half and place in prepared loaf pans. Sprinkle tops with cornmeal. Cover and let rise in a warm place until double in size (~45 minutes).
5. Preheat oven to 400°F. Bake about 25 minutes or until golden brown. Immediately remove from pans and cool on wire rack.

NUTRITION	
Serving size: 12 servings per loaf	Carbohydrates: 28 g
Each serving provides:	Sugar: 10 g
Calories: 135	Total fiber: 1.2 g
Total fat: 0.5 g	Protein: 4.5 g
Saturated fat: <1 g	Iron: 1.5 mg
Monounsaturated fat: <1 g	Magnesium: 15 mg
Polyunsaturated fat: <1 g	Calcium: 30 mg
Cholesterol: 1 mg	Vitamin A: 14 IU
Sodium: 148 mg	Vitamin C: <1 mg
Potassium: 152 mg	Vitamin D: <1 µg

SALADS

FlavorDoctor is especially delicious on salads to liven up the taste of greens and vegetables.

Cranberry Salad

YIELD: 8 SERVINGS

Ingredients

1 package (3 oz) raspberry Jell-O
1 can whole cranberry sauce (not jellied)
1 cup apple, peeled and chopped
1 cup celery, chopped
½ cup unsalted nuts

1. Mix Jell-O according to package directions.
2. When cool and the consistency of syrup, add cranberry sauce, apple, celery, and nuts.
3. Refrigerate until firm. Serve cold.

NUTRITION

Serving size: 1/2 cup	Carbohydrates: 17 g
Each serving provides:	Sugar: 13.5 g
Calories: 114	Total fiber: 1.3 g
Total fat: 4 g	Protein: 2.5 g
Saturated fat: <1 g	Iron: <1 mg
Monounsaturated fat: 1.1 g	Magnesium: 18 mg
Polyunsaturated fat: 2.8 g	Calcium: 11 mg
Cholesterol: 0 mg	Vitamin A: 28 IU
Sodium: 28 mg	Vitamin C: 1.1 mg
Potassium: 101 mg	Vitamin D: 0 µg

Mediterranean Pasta Salad

Ingredients

4 cups cooked small shell macaroni

1 tbsp olive oil

2 cups fresh green beans, cut into 1-inch pieces

½ cup lemon juice

⅓ cup olive oil

2 tsp dry mustard*

1 tbsp fresh parsley, chopped

1 tsp basil*

1 can (7¾ oz) water-packed tuna, drained

5 green onions, chopped

¼ tsp pepper*

1. Toss pasta with 1 tbsp olive oil in a bowl and set aside.
2. Blanch green beans by dropping into boiling water for 2 minutes. Transfer to a colander and chill under cold water. Drain.
3. In a large bowl, combine beans, lemon juice, ⅓ cup olive oil, mustard, parsley, and basil.
4. Add tuna, green onions, pasta, and pepper. Toss, then cover and chill at least 1 or 2 hours before serving.

NUTRITION

Serving size: 1½ cups	Carbohydrates: 34 g
Each serving provides:	Sugar: 1.8 g
Calories: 326	Total fiber: 3.5 g
Total fat: 14.5 g	Protein: 15 g
Saturated fat: 1 g	Iron: 2 mg
Monounsaturated fat: 4.5 g	Magnesium: 38 mg
Polyunsaturated fat: 9 g	Calcium: 42 mg
Cholesterol: 19 mg	Vitamin A: 470 IU
Sodium: 64 mg	Vitamin C: 18 mg
Potassium: 265 mg	Vitamin D: 0 µg

Roasted Vegetable Salad

Ingredients

12 new potatoes, halved

2 large red onions,
    each cut into 8 wedges

2 large yellow bell peppers,
    seeded and cubed

4 cloves garlic, peeled*

1 eggplant, thickly sliced

1 tsp fresh rosemary, chopped

2 tsp fresh thyme, chopped*

2 tbsp olive oil

1 pint cherry tomatoes, halved

⅓ cup toasted pine nuts

1 bag (10 oz) baby spinach leaves

2 tbsp balsamic vinegar

1. Preheat oven to 400° F. Line a baking sheet with aluminum foil.
2. Place potatoes in a microwave-safe dish, and place in the microwave. Cook on high until the potatoes are just tender, 3 to 4 minutes.
3. Place the potatoes in a large bowl along with the onion, bell pepper, garlic, and eggplant. Sprinkle with rosemary, thyme, and olive oil. Toss to coat the vegetables with olive oil. You can add a sodium-free seasoning to taste (such as Mrs. Dash). Spread vegetables onto prepared baking sheet.
4. Roast the vegetables in the preheated oven until they begin to brown at the edges, about 35 minutes. Stir in the cherry tomato halves, and continue cooking 15 minutes more.
5. Toss the roasted vegetables in a large bowl with the pine nuts, spinach, and balsamic vinegar.

NUTRITION

Each serving provides:

Calories: 215

Total fat: 9.5 g
    Saturated fat: 1 g
    Monounsaturated fat 3.5 g
    Polyunsaturated fat: 5 g

Cholesterol: 0 mg

Sodium: 67 mg

Potassium: 982 mg

Carbohydrates: 26 g
    Sugar: 6.8 g
    Total fiber: 8 g

Protein: 6.5 g

Iron: 5 mg

Magnesium: 112 mg

Calcium: 74 mg

Vitamin A: 2,912 IU

Vitamin C: 141 mg

Vitamin D: 0 μg

Cucumber Couscous Salad

Ingredients

10 ounces uncooked couscous

2 tbsp olive oil

½ cup lemon juice

¼ tsp salt

½ tsp ground black pepper*

1 cucumber, seeded and chopped

½ cup finely chopped green onions

½ cup fresh parsley, chopped

¼ cup fresh basil, chopped*

8 leaves lettuce

8 slices lemon

1. In a medium saucepan, bring 1¾ cups water to a boil. Stir in couscous; cover. Remove from heat; let stand, covered, 5 minutes. Cool to room temperature.

2. Meanwhile, in a medium bowl combine oil, lemon juice, salt, and pepper. Stir in cucumber, green onion, parsley, basil, and couscous. Mix well and chill for at least 1 hour.

3. Line a plate with lettuce leaves. Spoon couscous mixture over leaves and garnish with lemon wedges.

NUTRITION	
Each serving provides:	Carbohydrates: 32 g
Calories: 186	Sugar: 8 g
Total fat: 4 g	Total fiber: 3.5 g
Saturated fat: 1 g	Protein: 5.5 g
Monounsaturated fat: 2.5 g	Iron: 2 mg
Polyunsaturated fat: 0.5 g	Magnesium: 31 mg
Cholesterol: 0 mg	Calcium: 78 mg
Sodium: 44 mg	Vitamin A: 59 IU
Potassium: 336 mg	Vitamin C: 23 mg
	Vitamin D: 0 µg

Balsamic Vinaigrette Pasta Salad

Ingredients

3 cups pasta of your choice (8 ounces)

2 cups yellow summer squash, sliced

1 cup green peas

½ red sweet pepper, sliced

1 can (6 oz) pitted black olives, drained and chopped

1 cup cherry tomatoes, halved

½ cup red onion, chopped

2 tsp dried basil, crushed*

1 cup balsamic vinaigrette

1. Cook pasta and drain. Rinse with cold water; drain again.
2. In a large bowl, combine all ingredients and toss gently to coat.
3. Chill and cover for 2 to 24 hours.

NUTRITION

Each serving provides:	
Calories: 155	Carbohydrates: 32 g
Total fat: 1 g	Sugar: 4 g
Saturated fat: <1 g	Total fiber: 3.5 g
Monounsaturated fat: <1 g	Protein: 4.5 g
Polyunsaturated fat: <1 g	Iron: 2 mg
Cholesterol: 0 mg	Magnesium: 35 mg
Sodium: 51 mg	Calcium: 54 mg
Potassium: 278 mg	Vitamin A: 105 IU
	Vitamin C: 29 mg
	Vitamin D: 0 µg

Blue Cheese and Pear Salad

Ingredients

¼ cup sugar

½ cup pecans

⅓ cup olive oil

3 tbsp red wine vinegar

1½ tsp sugar

1½ tsp mustard

1 clove garlic, chopped

¼ teaspoon light salt

Fresh ground black pepper to taste

1 head leaf lettuce, torn into bite-size pieces

3 pears, peeled, cored, and chopped

3 ounces blue cheese, crumbled

½ cup thinly sliced green onions

1. In a skillet over medium heat, stir ¼ cup of sugar together with the pecans. Continue stirring gently until sugar has melted and caramelizes the pecans. Carefully transfer nuts onto waxed paper. Allow to cool, and break into pieces.

2. For the dressing, blend oil, vinegar, 1½ teaspoons sugar, mustard, chopped garlic, salt, and pepper.

3. In a large serving bowl, layer lettuce, pears, blue cheese, avocado, and green onions. Pour dressing over salad, sprinkle with pecans, and serve.

NUTRITION

Each serving provides:	
Calories: 230	Carbohydrates: 19 g
Total fat: 15.5 g	Sugar: 4 g
Saturated fat: 3.5 g	Total fiber: 2 g
Monounsaturated fat: 10 g	Protein: 3.5 g
Polyunsaturated fat: 2 g	Iron: 0.5 mg
Cholesterol: 8 mg	Magnesium: 19 mg
Sodium: 208 mg	Calcium: 77 mg
Potassium: 258 mg	Vitamin A: 48.5 IU
	Vitamin C: 5.5 mg
	Vitamin D: 0 µg

Caribbean Sweet Potato Salad

Ingredients

2 large sweet potatoes, peeled and quartered

1 cup corn

1 tsp Dijon-style mustard

2 tbsp fresh lime juice

3 tbsp fresh cilantro, chopped

1 clove garlic, minced

3 tbsp canola oil

⅛ tsp salt

¼ tsp ground black pepper

1 cucumber, halved lengthwise and chopped

½ red onion, thinly sliced

¼ cup finely chopped peanuts

1. Place the potato pieces in a large saucepan, and cover with water. Bring to a boil, turn the heat down, and simmer for 10 to 15 minutes. Remove a piece of potato, and cut it in half to see if it is cooked enough. Once the potatoes are tender, add corn kernels; cook another 30 seconds. Drain through a colander. Fill the saucepan with cold water, and place vegetables into water. Cool for 5 minutes, and drain.

2. In a large bowl, whisk together mustard, lime juice, cilantro, and garlic. Slowly whisk in oil. Mix in salt and black pepper.

3. Cut cooled potatoes into 1-inch cubes, and add to dressing along with cucumber and red onion. Toss well. Serve at room temperature or chilled. Toss the peanuts in just before serving.

NUTRITION	
Each serving provides:	Carbohydrates: 20 g
Calories: 184	Sugar: 3 g
Total fat: 10 g	Total fiber: 2 g
Saturated fat: 1 g	Protein: 3.5 g
Monounsaturated fat: 5.5 g	Iron: 0.5 mg
Polyunsaturated fat: 3.5 g	Magnesium: 35 mg
Cholesterol: 0 mg	Calcium: 22 mg
Sodium: 53 mg	Vitamin A: 866 IU
Potassium: 242 mg	Vitamin C: 12 mg
	Vitamin D: 0 µg

Summary Corn and Tomato Salad

Ingredients

¼ cup fresh basil, minced

3 tbsp olive oil

2 tsp lime juice

1 tsp sugar

¼ tsp salt

¼ tsp pepper*

2 cups frozen corn, thawed

2 cups cherry tomatoes, halved

1 cup chopped, seeded, peeled cucumber

1. In a jar with a tight-fitting lid, combine the basil, oil, lime juice, sugar, salt, and pepper; shake well.
2. In a large bowl, combine the corn, tomatoes, and cucumber. Drizzle with dressing and toss to coat. Refrigerate until serving.

NUTRITION	
Each serving provides:	Carbohydrates: 25 g
Calories: 209	Sugar: 7 g
Total fat: 10.5 g	Total fiber: 5 g
Saturated fat: 1.5 g	Protein: 3.5 g
Monounsaturated fat: 7.5 g	Iron: 2.5 mg
Polyunsaturated fat: 1.5 g	Magnesium: 46 mg
Cholesterol: 0 mg	Calcium: 105 mg
Sodium: 87 mg	Vitamin A: 116 IU
Potassium: 586 mg	Vitamin C: 25 mg
	Vitamin D: 0 µg

Pecan and Avocado Salad

YIELD: 1 SERVING

Ingredients

1 cup baby spinach leaves

1 tablespoon dried cranberries

1 tablespoon chopped pecans

½ apple, cored and diced

1 tablespoon diced red onion

2 tablespoons grated carrot

¼ avocado, peeled and diced

1 tablespoon balsamic vinaigrette salad dressing, or to taste

1. Place spinach, cranberries, pecans, apple, onion, carrot, and avocado into a bowl. Drizzle with balsamic vinaigrette, and toss to coat.

NUTRITION

Each serving provides:	
Calories: 253	Carbohydrates: 34 g
Total fat: 11.5 g	Sugar: 10 g
Saturated fat: 1.6 g	Total fiber: 8 g
Monounsaturated fat: 7.7 g	Protein: 3.5 g
Polyunsaturated fat: 2.2 g	Iron: 2.5 mg
Cholesterol: 0 mg	Magnesium: 79 mg
Sodium: 58 mg	Calcium: 78 mg
Potassium: 808 mg	Vitamin A: 795 IU
	Vitamin C: 27 mg
	Vitamin D: 0 µg

Glazed Parsnip Salad with Pecans

YIELD: 6 SERVINGS

Ingredients

2½ cups parsnip, cut into thin strips
2½ cups carrot, cut into thin strips
½ cup broccoli stems, cut into thin strips
¾ cup orange juice
⅓ cup dried cranberries
½ tsp ground ginger
2 pears, firm, peeled and sliced
⅓ cup pecan halves
3 tbsp packed brown sugar
2 tbsp margarine

1. In a large skillet, combine the first 6 ingredients. Bring to a boil, then reduce heat to medium. Cook, uncovered, for ~6 to 8 minutes, stirring occasionally. (Most of the liquid should evaporate.)
2. Stir in pears, pecans, brown sugar, and margarine. Cook, uncovered, for another 2 to 3 minutes, or until vegetables are glazed.

NUTRITION	
Each serving provides:	Carbohydrates: 42 g
Calories: 325	Sugar: 12 g
Total fat: 5.5 g	Total fiber: 6.5 g
Saturated fat: 0.75 g	Protein: 2.7 g
Monounsaturated fat: 3 g	Iron: 1.2 mg
Polyunsaturated fat: 1.8 g	Magnesium: 46 mg
Cholesterol: 0 mg	Calcium: 62 mg
Sodium: 54 mg	Vitamin A: 1,346 IU
Potassium: 611 mg	Vitamin C: 49 mg
	Vitamin D: 0 µg

SOUPS

Minestrone

Ingredients

¼ cup olive oil

1 clove garlic, minced
(or ⅛ tsp powder)*

1⅓ cups onion, coarsely chopped

1½ cups celery with leaves,
coarsely chopped

1 can (6 oz) tomato paste
(no added salt)

1 tbsp fresh parsley, chopped

1 cup carrots, sliced, fresh or frozen

4¾ cups cabbage, shredded

1 can (1 lb) tomatoes, cut up

1 cup canned red kidney beans,
drained, rinsed

1½ cups frozen green peas

1½ cups fresh green beans

Dash hot sauce

11 cups water

2 cups spaghetti, uncooked, broken

1. Heat oil in 4-quart saucepan. Add garlic, onion, and celery, and sauté for about 5 minutes.
2. Add all remaining ingredients except spaghetti. Stir until ingredients are well mixed.
3. Bring to boil and reduce heat, cover, and simmer for about 45 minutes or until vegetables are tender.
4. Add uncooked spaghetti and simmer for only 2 to 3 minutes.

NUTRITION

Each serving provides:	
Calories: 115	Carbohydrates: 23 g
Total fat: 0.5 g	Sugar: 7 g
Saturated fat: 0 g	Total fiber: 5 g
Monounsaturated fat: 0.5 g	Protein: 5 g
Polyunsaturated fat: 0 g	Iron: 2 mg
Cholesterol: 0 mg	Magnesium: 32 mg
Sodium: 189 mg	Calcium: 62 mg
Potassium: 467 mg	Vitamin A: 1,259 IU
	Vitamin C: 26 mg
	Vitamin D: 0 µg

Turkey Soup with Barley

YIELD: 8 TO 10 SERVINGS

Ingredients

6 pounds turkey breast with bones
  (with at least 2 cups meat)
2 medium onions
3 stalks celery
1 tsp dried thyme*
½ tsp dried rosemary

½ tsp dried sage*
1 tsp dried basil*
½ tsp dried marjoram
½ tsp dried tarragon
Black pepper to taste*
1½ cups barley

1. Place turkey breast in large 6-quart pot. Cover with water until at least three-quarters full.
2. Peel onions, cut into large pieces, and add to pot. Wash celery stalks, slice, and add to pot.
3. Simmer, covered, for about 2½ hours.
4. Remove carcass from pot. Divide soup into smaller, shallower containers for quick cooling in refrigerator.
5. After cooling, skim off fat.
6. While soup cools, remove remaining meat from turkey carcass. Cut into pieces.
7. Add turkey meat to skimmed soup, along with herbs and spices.
8. Bring to boil and add barley. Continue cooking on low boil for about 20 minutes, until barley is done. Serve at once or refrigerate for later reheating.

NUTRITION	
Each serving provides:	Carbohydrates: 27 g
Calories: 236	Sugar: 5 g
Total fat: 2.5 g	Total fiber: 5.5 g
Saturated fat: 1.5 g	Protein: 26 g
Monounsaturated fat: <1 g	Iron: 2.3 mg
Polyunsaturated fat: 1 g	Magnesium: 50 mg
Cholesterol: 59 mg	Calcium: 44 mg
Sodium: 68 mg	Vitamin A: 3 IU
Potassium: 407 mg	Vitamin C: 3 mg
	Vitamin D: 0 µg

San Francisco Cioppino

YIELD: 8 SERVINGS

Ingredients

¼ cup olive oil

1 onion, chopped

4 cloves garlic, minced*

1 green bell pepper, chopped

1 fresh red chili pepper, seeded and chopped*

½ cup chopped fresh parsley

Salt, to taste

Pepper to taste*

2 tsp dried basil*

1 tsp dried oregano

1 tsp dried thyme

1 can (28 oz) low-sodium crushed tomatoes

1 can (8 oz) low-sodium tomato sauce

½ cup water

1 pinch paprika

1 pinch cayenne pepper

1 can (10 oz) minced clams, drained with juice reserved

1 cup white wine

25 mussels, cleaned and debearded

25 shrimp

10 ounces scallops

1 pound cod fillets, cubed

1. In a large pot over medium heat, heat the olive oil, and sauté the onion, garlic, bell pepper, and chili pepper until tender.
2. Add parsley, salt and pepper, basil, oregano, thyme, tomatoes, tomato sauce, water, paprika, cayenne pepper, and juice from the clams.
3. Stir well, reduce heat, and simmer 1 to 2 hours, adding wine a little at a time.

(continued)

San Francisco Cioppino (*continued*)

4. About 10 minutes before serving, add clams, mussels, shrimp, scallops, and cod.
5. Turn the heat up slightly and stir. When the seafood is cooked through (the mussels will have opened, the shrimp turned pink, and the cod will be flaky), serve your delicious cioppino.

NUTRITION

Each serving provides:	Carbohydrates: 16 g
Calories: 260	Sugar: 4 g
Total fat: 7.1 g	Total fiber: 3.3 g
Saturated fat: 1.1 g	Protein: 33 g
Monounsaturated fat: 4 g	Iron: 16 mg
Polyunsaturated fat: 2 g	Magnesium: 98 mg
Cholesterol: 92 mg	Calcium: mg
Sodium: 278 mg	Vitamin A: 402 IU
Potassium: 1012 mg	Vitamin C: 61 mg
	Vitamin D: 7.5 µg

Cuban Black Bean Soup

YIELD: 4 SERVINGS

Ingredients

1 pound dried black beans, rinsed and soaked overnight

1½ cups low-sodium vegetable broth

1 cup chunky salsa

1 tsp ground cumin*

4 tbsp low-fat sour cream

2 tbsp green onion, thinly sliced

1. In an electric food processor or blender, combine beans, broth, salsa, and cumin. Blend until fairly smooth.
2. Heat the bean mixture in a saucepan over medium heat until thoroughly heated.
3. Ladle soup into 4 individual bowls, and top each bowl with 1 tablespoon of the sour cream and ½ tablespoon green onions.

NUTRITION	
Each serving provides:	Carbohydrates: 33 g
Calories: 204	Sugar: 1.2 g
Total fat: 2.2 g	Total fiber: 12.9 g
Saturated fat: 1.2 g	Protein: 13 g
Monounsaturated fat: 0.5 g	Iron: 2.5 mg
Polyunsaturated fat: 0.5 g	Magnesium: 80 mg
Cholesterol: 5 mg	Calcium: 53 mg
Sodium: 388 mg	Vitamin A: 34 IU
Potassium: 176 mg	Vitamin C: 5 mg
	Vitamin D: 0 µg

Corn Chowder

Ingredients

1 tbsp vegetable oil

2 tbsp celery, finely diced

2 tbsp onion, finely diced

2 tbsp green pepper, finely diced

1 package (10 oz) frozen whole kernel corn

1 cup ½-inch raw potatoes, peeled and diced

1 cup water

¼ tsp salt

Black pepper to taste

¼ tsp paprika*

2 cups low-fat (1%) or skim milk

2 tbsp flour

2 tbsp fresh parsley, chopped

1. Heat oil in medium saucepan.
2. Add celery, onion, and green pepper and sauté for 2 minutes.
3. Add corn, potatoes, water, salt, pepper, and paprika. Bring to a boil; reduce heat to medium; and cook, covered, about 10 minutes or until potatoes are tender.
4. Place ½ cup milk in a jar with tight-fitting lid. Add flour and shake vigorously.
5. Add gradually to cooked vegetables and add remaining milk.
6. Cook, stirring constantly, until mixture comes to a boil and thickens. Serve garnished with chopped fresh parsley.

NUTRITION	
Each serving provides:	Carbohydrates: 30 g
Calories: 180	Sugar: 4 g
Total fat: 3.5 g	Total fiber: 2.7 g
Saturated fat: 0.5 g	Protein: 7 g
Monounsaturated fat: 0.5 g	Iron: 0.8 mg
Polyunsaturated fat: 2.5 g	Magnesium: 38 mg
Cholesterol: 2.2 mg	Calcium: mg
Sodium: 146 mg	Vitamin A: 111 IU
Potassium: 577 mg	Vitamin C: 13 mg
	Vitamin D: 1.2 µg

New Orleans Chicken Gumbo with Okra

Ingredients

8 cups water

1 tsp garlic powder

1 tbsp hot pepper sauce

2 carrots, sliced thin

4 ounces fresh mushrooms

1 package (10 oz) frozen okra, thawed and sliced

¼ cup uncooked wild rice

1 skinless, boneless chicken breast half, cut into cubes

1½ cups uncooked pasta (rotini)

Salt to taste

Ground black pepper to taste*

3 green onions, sliced thin

1. Bring the water to a boil. Add the garlic powder and the hot pepper sauce. Put the carrots and mushrooms into the pot of water. Cook for 5 minutes.

2. Add the okra, wild rice, and chicken cubes. Turn heat to low, and cook for 3 hours.

3. Add the spiral pasta, and cook for 10 minutes. Add salt and pepper to taste. Serve hot, garnished with green onions.

NUTRITION	
Each serving provides:	Carbohydrates:24 g
Calories: 142	Sugar: 3 g
Total fat: 1.5 g	Total fiber: 2.5 g
Saturated fat: 0.5 g	Protein: 8 g
Monounsaturated fat: 0.5 g	Iron: 1.8 mg
Polyunsaturated fat: 0.5 g	Magnesium: 55 mg
Cholesterol: 9 mg	Calcium: 103 mg
Sodium: 74 mg	Vitamin A: 535 IU
Potassium: 289 mg	Vitamin C: 7.7 mg
	Vitamin D: 0.3 µg

Lentil Soup

YIELD: 8 SERVINGS

Ingredients

¼ cup olive oil

1 onion, chopped

2 carrots, diced

2 stalks celery, chopped

2 cloves garlic, minced

1 tsp dried oregano*

1 bay leaf* *(to be removed after cooking)*

1 tsp dried basil

2 cups dry lentils

8 cups water

1 can (14.5 oz) crushed tomatoes (no added salt)

½ cup spinach, rinsed and thinly sliced

2 tbsp vinegar

Salt to taste

Ground black pepper to taste

1. In a large soup pot, heat oil over medium heat. Add onions, carrots, and celery; cook and stir until onion is tender. Stir in garlic, oregano, bay leaf, and basil; cook for 2 minutes.
2. Stir in lentils, and add water and tomatoes. Bring to a boil. Reduce heat, and simmer for at least 1 hour.
3. When ready to serve, stir in spinach, and cook until it wilts. Stir in vinegar, and season to taste with salt and pepper, and more vinegar if desired.

NUTRITION	
Each serving provides:	Carbohydrates: 29 g
Calories: 247	Sugar: 5 g
Total fat: 6.5 g	Total fiber: 5 g
Saturated fat: 1 g	Protein: 18 g
Monounsaturated fat: 5 g	Iron: 12 mg
Polyunsaturated fat: 0.5 g	Calcium: 110 mg
Cholesterol: 0 mg	Vitamin A: 566 IU
Sodium: 97 mg	Vitamin C: 15.5 mg
Potassium: 330 mg	Vitamin D: 0 µg

Crab and Roasted Corn Soup

Ingredients

1 package (16 oz) frozen whole-kernel corn

2 cups chopped onion (2 large)

1½ cups red sweet pepper, coarsely chopped (3 medium)

1 tbsp canola oil

4 cans (14 oz each) low-sodium chicken broth

½ tsp dried thyme, crushed*

⅛ tsp cayenne pepper*

⅓ cup all-purpose flour

½ cup low-fat sour cream

4 ounces cooked crabmeat, cut into bite-size pieces (⅔ cup)

1. Preheat oven to 450°F. Thaw frozen corn. Pat dry with paper towels. Line baking pan with foil; lightly grease foil. Spread corn in prepared pan. Bake in oven for 10 minutes; stir. Bake for another 10 minutes until golden brown, stirring once or twice. Remove from oven; set aside.

2. In a Dutch oven, cook onion and sweet pepper in hot oil over medium heat for 3 to 4 minutes or until nearly tender. Add roasted corn, 3 cans of broth, thyme, and cayenne pepper. Bring to a boil, then reduce to a simmer, uncovered, for 15 minutes.

3. In a large screw-top jar, combine remaining can of broth and the flour. Cover and shake well. Stir into soup. Cook and stir until slightly thickened and bubbly. Stir for 1 minute more and then stir in the sour cream; heat through.

4. To serve, ladle soup into bowls and divide crabmeat among bowls.

NUTRITION	
Each serving provides:	Carbohydrates: 30 g
Calories: 200	Sugar: 5 g
Total fat: 4.4 g	Total fiber: 4 g
Saturated fat: 1.7 g	Protein: 10 g
Monounsaturated fat: 1.7 g	Iron: 11 mg
Polyunsaturated fat: 1 g	Magnesium: 34 mg
Cholesterol: 25 mg	Calcium: 73 mg
Sodium: 370 mg	Vitamin A: 270 IU
Potassium: 410 mg	Vitamin C: 77 mg
	Vitamin D: 0 µg

VEGETABLES / SIDE DISHES

Green Beans with
Slivered Almonds, Garlic, and Basil

YIELD: 4 SERVINGS

Ingredients

1½ pounds fresh green beans, trimmed

⅓ cup green onions, sliced

1 garlic clove, minced

2 tsp olive oil

¼ cup balsamic vinegar

4 tsp sugar

1½ tsp minced fresh basil*

⅛ tsp salt

¼ cup sliced almonds, toasted

1. Place beans in a saucepan and cover with water. Bring to a boil; cook, uncovered, for 8 to 10 minutes or until tender.

2. Meanwhile, in a nonstick skillet, sauté onions and garlic in oil until onions are tender. Add the vinegar, sugar, basil, and salt. Bring to a boil; cook until liquid is reduced by half.

3. Drain beans; add to onion mixture. Cook and stir until heated through.

4. Sprinkle with almonds.

NUTRITION	
Each serving provides:	Carbohydrates: 24 g
Calories: 159	Sugar: 2 g
Total fat: 5 g	Total fiber: 6 g
Saturated fat: 0.5 g	Protein: 4.5 g
Monounsaturated fat: 3.5 g	Iron: 2.8 mg
Polyunsaturated fat: 1 g	Magnesium: 63 mg
Cholesterol: 0 mg	Calcium: 110 mg
Sodium: 46 mg	Vitamin A: 118 IU
Potassium: 635 mg	Vitamin C: 20 mg
	Vitamin D: 0 µg

Moroccan Couscous Pilaf

Ingredients

1 tbsp olive oil

1 tbsp unsalted butter

1 small onion, cut into ¼-inch dice

¾ tsp ground cumin*

Pinch of cayenne pepper

1 box (10 oz) medium-grain couscous

¼ tsp salt

¼ tsp freshly ground pepper*

2 tbsp fresh flat-leaf parsley, coarsely chopped

1. Bring 2¼ cups water to a boil in a medium saucepan.
2. Meanwhile, in a large saucepan, heat olive oil and butter over medium-low heat. Add onions and cook until lightly browned, about 8 minutes. Stir in cumin and cayenne pepper, and sauté for 1 minute more.
3. Stir in couscous, salt, pepper, and boiling water. Cover and simmer over low heat until tender and water is absorbed, about 10 minutes. Add parsley and serve.

NUTRITION	
Each serving provides:	Carbohydrates: 38 g
Calories: 217	Sugar: 10 g
Total fat: 4.5 g	Total fiber: 2.5 g
Saturated fat: 1.5 g	Protein: 6 g
Monounsaturated fat: 2.2 g	Iron: 0.5 mg
Polyunsaturated fat: <1 g	Magnesium: 24 mg
Cholesterol: 5 mg	Calcium: 18 mg
Sodium: 55 mg	Vitamin A: 26 IU
Potassium: 184 mg	Vitamin C: 3 mg
	Vitamin D: 0 µg

Autumn Succotash

Ingredients

1 package (10 oz) frozen lima beans
1 package (10 oz) frozen whole-kernel corn
2 small tomatoes, seeded and chopped
¼ cup green onion, sliced
1 tbsp fresh parsley, snipped
¼ cup red wine vinegar
2 tbsp Italian salad dressing
¼ tsp dry mustard*

1. Cook lima beans and corn according to package directions; drain. In a bowl, combine lima beans, corn, tomato, green onion, and parsley.
2. In a small mixing bowl whisk together red wine vinegar, dressing, and mustard. Pour over lima bean mixture; toss to coat. Serve at room temperature or chilled.

NUTRITION

Serving size: 1/2 cup
Each serving provides:
Calories: 119
Total fat: 3 g
  Saturated fat: 0.5 g
  Monounsaturated fat: 1 g
  Polyunsaturated fat: 1.5 g
Cholesterol: 0 mg
Sodium: 30 mg
Potassium: 332 mg

Carbohydrates: 19 g
  Sugar: 4 g
  Total fiber: 4 g
Protein: 4 g
Iron: 1 mg
Magnesium: 28 mg
Calcium: 17 mg
Vitamin A: 38 IU
Vitamin C: 14 mg
Vitamin D: 0 µg

Mediterranean Orzo Pasta

Ingredients

3 quarts water

1⅓ cups (8 oz) dry orzo pasta

2 tsp olive oil

1 clove garlic, minced

½ tsp Italian seasoning (blend of marjoram, thyme, rosemary, savory, sage, oregano, and basil)

1 tbsp Parmesan cheese, grated

1. Bring water to boil. Add orzo to water and stir. Return to a boil and cook, uncovered, for 9 to 11 minutes or until done (avoid overcooking for best results).
2. Remove from heat and drain well in colander.
3. Pour drained pasta into serving bowl. Add olive oil, garlic, Italian seasoning, and Parmesan cheese. Toss gently and serve.

NUTRITION	
Each serving provides:	Carbohydrates: 25 g
Calories: 128	Sugar: 8 g
Total fat: 2 g	Total fiber: 0.5 g
Saturated fat: 0.5 g	Protein: 2.5 g
Monounsaturated fat: 1.25 g	Iron: 1.1 mg
Polyunsaturated fat: <1 g	Magnesium: 10.5 mg
Cholesterol: 0.8 mg	Calcium: 35 mg
Sodium: 21 mg	Vitamin A: 2.6 IU
Potassium: 42 mg	Vitamin C: <1 mg
	Vitamin D: 0 µg

Broccoli-Cauliflower-Carrot Bake

Ingredients

3 cups broccoli, raw

2 cups cauliflower, raw

1 cup frozen whole small onions or 3 medium onions, quartered

1 cup carrots, chopped

4 tbsp butter

2 tbsp flour

¼ tsp black pepper*

1 cup fat-free milk

1 package (3 oz) cream cheese, softened

½ cup sharp cheddar cheese, shredded

½ cup soft breadcrumbs

1. Wash and cut vegetables; steam until crisp but tender. Drain.

2. In saucepan, melt 2 tbsp of the butter; blend in flour and pepper. Add milk and cook/stir until bubbly and thick.

3. Reduce heat and blend in cream cheese until smooth.

4. Place vegetables in 1½-quart casserole dish and pour sauce over and mix lightly. Top with shredded cheese.

5. Bake for 15 minutes at 350°F.

6. Meanwhile, mix the breadcrumbs and remaining butter and then sprinkle on casserole and bake for an additional 25 minutes.

NUTRITION

Each serving provides:	
Calories: 132	Carbohydrates: 11 g
Total fat: 7.5 g	Sugar: <1 g
Saturated fat: 4.5 g	Total fiber: 2 g
Monounsaturated fat: 2.3 g	Protein: 5 g
Polyunsaturated fat: <1 g	Iron: 1 mg
Cholesterol: 21 mg	Magnesium: 19 mg
Sodium: 163 mg	Calcium: 193 mg
Potassium: 260 mg	Vitamin A: 455 IU
	Vitamin C: 31 mg
	Vitamin D: 0.5 µg

Roasted Sweet Potatoes

YIELD: 6 SERVINGS

Ingredients

2 large sweet potatoes, peeled and cut into 1-inch chunks

2 medium Vidalia or other sweet onions, cut into 1-inch chunks

3 tbsp olive oil

¼ cup amaretto liqueur

1 tsp dried thyme

Freshly ground black pepper to taste*

¼ cup sliced almonds, toasted

1. Heat oven to 425°F.
2. Toss first 6 ingredients in a shallow medium-size baking dish.
3. Cover; bake 30 minutes. Uncover; bake for an additional 20 minutes.
4. Sprinkle with almonds

NUTRITION

Each serving provides:	
Calories: 159	Carbohydrates: 18 g
Total fat: 8.5 g	Sugar: 6 g
Saturated fat: 1.2 g	Total fiber: 2 g
Monounsaturated fat: 6.1 g	Protein: 2.5 g
Polyunsaturated fat: 1.2 g	Iron: 0.5 mg
Cholesterol: 0 mg	Magnesium: 22.5 mg
Sodium: 10 mg	Calcium: 32.5 mg
Potassium: 211 mg	Vitamin A: 858 IU
	Vitamin C: 13 mg
	Vitamin D: 0 µg

Roasted Acorn Squash

Ingredients

1 medium acorn squash, halved and seeded

1 tbsp butter

2 tbsp brown sugar

1. Preheat oven to 350°F.
2. Turn acorn squash upside down onto a cookie sheet. Bake in a 350°F oven until it begins to soften, approximately 30 to 45 minutes.
3. Remove squash from the oven and turn onto a plate so that the flesh is facing upward. Place butter and brown sugar into the squash, and place remaining squash over the other piece. Place squash in a baking dish (so the squash won't slide around too much) while baking.
4. Place squash in the 350°F oven and bake another 30 minutes.

NUTRITION

Each serving provides:	
Calories: 262	Carbohydrates: 49 g
Total fat: 6 g	Sugar: 12 g
Saturated fat: 3.5 g	Total fiber: 10.5 g
Monounsaturated fat: 1.7 g	Protein: 3 g
Polyunsaturated fat: <1 g	Iron: 2.5 mg
Cholesterol: 15 mg	Magnesium: 109 mg
Sodium: 73 mg	Calcium: 121 mg
Potassium: 1,120 mg	Vitamin A: 159 IU
	Vitamin C: 26 mg
	Vitamin D: 0 µg

Crispy Edamame

Ingredients

1 package (12 oz) frozen edamame (green soybeans)
1 tbsp olive oil
¼ cup Parmesan cheese, grated
Pepper to taste*

1. Preheat oven to 400°F.
2. Thaw edamame under cold water in a colander. Drain.
3. Spread edamame beans into bottom of a 9-by-13-inch baking dish and drizzle with olive oil. Sprinkle cheese over top and season with pepper.
4. Bake until cheese is crispy and golden (~15 minutes).

NUTRITION

Each serving provides:	
Calories: 106	Carbohydrates: 5 g
Total fat: 6 g	Sugar: <1 g
Saturated fat: 1.3 g	Total fiber: 2.5 g
Monounsaturated fat: 2.4 g	Protein: 8 g
Polyunsaturated fat: 2.3 g	Iron: 2.2 mg
Cholesterol: 2.5 mg	Magnesium: 38 mg
Sodium: 59 mg	Calcium: 86 mg
Potassium: 223 mg	Vitamin A: 5.8 IU
	Vitamin C: 0.7 mg
	Vitamin D: 0 µg

Summer Vegetable Ratatouille

Ingredients

2 tbsp olive oil

2 medium onions, chopped

3 cloves garlic, minced

1 medium eggplant, cubed

1 zucchini, cubed

1 medium yellow squash, cubed

1 green bell pepper, seeded and cubed

1 yellow bell pepper, seeded and cubed

1 red bell pepper, seeded and cubed

2 cups tomatoes, chopped

½ cup dry white wine

Pepper to taste*

½ tbsp dried oregano*

2 tbsp fresh basil, chopped*

1. Heat oil in a large skillet over medium-low heat. Add the onions and garlic and cook until tender.
2. Stir in the eggplant, zucchini, squash, bell peppers, tomatoes, wine, and black pepper. Bring to a boil; reduce heat. Simmer, covered, about 10 minutes or until vegetables are tender.
3. Uncover and cook for another 5 minutes or until most of the liquid has evaporated, stirring occasionally. Season to taste with additional black pepper.
4. Stir in fresh basil just before serving.

NUTRITION	
Each serving provides:	Carbohydrates: 10.5 g
Calories: 80	Sugar: <1 g
Total fat: 3.5 g	Total fiber: 3 g
Saturated fat: 0.5 g	Protein: 1.5 g
Monounsaturated fat: 2.5 g	Iron: 1.3 mg
Polyunsaturated fat: 0.5 g	Magnesium: 25 mg
Cholesterol: 0 mg	Calcium: 50 mg
Sodium: 97 mg	Vitamin A: 205 IU
Potassium: 360 mg	Vitamin C: 66 mg
	Vitamin D: 0 µg

Tabbouleh

YIELD: 12 SERVINGS

Ingredients

2 cups cracked wheat (bulgur)
2 cups very hot water
1 cucumber, chopped
2 small tomatoes, chopped
1 bunch green onions (8), sliced
½ cup fresh chopped mint
2 cups fresh chopped parsley
1 clove garlic, minced (optional)
½ cup fresh lemon juice
¾ cup extra virgin olive oil
1 tbsp pepper
⅛ tsp salt

1. Soak the cracked wheat in the hot water until the water is absorbed, about 30 minutes. Drain any excess water, if necessary, and squeeze dry.
2. In a medium bowl, combine wheat, cucumber, tomatoes, green onions, mint, parsley, and garlic.
3. In a separate bowl, mix lemon juice, oil, pepper and salt together and stir into the salad mixture.
4. Serve chilled or at room temperature.

NUTRITION	
Each serving provides:	Carbohydrates: 22 g
Calories: 230	Sugar: 9 g
Total fat: 14 g	Total fiber: 5.5 g
Saturated fat: 2 g	Protein: 4 g
Monounsaturated fat: 10.5 g	Iron: 1.8 mg
Polyunsaturated fat: 1.5 g	Magnesium: 50 mg
Cholesterol: 0 mg	Calcium: 38 mg
Sodium: 25 mg	Vitamin A: 76 IU
Potassium: 313 mg	Vitamin C: 30 mg
	Vitamin D: 0 µg

ENTRÉES

Polynesian Turkey Kabobs

YIELD: 15 SERVINGS

Ingredients

1 pound lean ground turkey, raw

⅓ cup unsalted crackers, crushed (5 crackers)

¼ cup liquid egg substitute

¼ cup onion, chopped

1 tsp ground ginger*

1 garlic clove, crushed

1 can (20 oz) pineapple chunks in juice, drained

1 large red bell pepper

1 large green bell pepper

⅓ cup reserved pineapple juice

2 tbsp margarine, melted

2 tbsp orange marmalade

1½ tsp ground ginger*

1. In a medium bowl, mix first six ingredients. Shape into meatballs.
2. Arrange meatballs on fifteen 8-inch skewers with pineapple chunks and pepper pieces and place on broiler pan.
3. In a small bowl, stir pineapple juice, margarine, marmalade, and ginger until blended. Brush over kabobs.
4. Broil 4 inches from heat source for 20 minutes, turning once and basting with sauce.

NUTRITION	
Each serving provides:	Carbohydrates: 9.9 g
Calories: 90	Sugar: 7 g
Total fat: 2 g	Total fiber: 1 g
Saturated fat: 0.8 g	Protein: 8 g
Monounsaturated fat: 0.5 g	Iron: 0.87 mg
Polyunsaturated fat: 0.7 g	Magnesium: 5.37 mg
Cholesterol: 21.5 mg	Calcium: 23 mg
Sodium: 73 mg	Vitamin A: 599.05 IU
Potassium: 110 mg	Vitamin C: 35.8 mg
	Vitamin D: 0 µg

Spinach Lasagna

Ingredients

1 yellow onion, chopped

2 cans (14.5 oz each) whole tomatoes (no added salt), chopped

2 cans (6 oz each) tomato paste (low sodium)

2 cups water

1 tbsp parsley, chopped

1 tsp salt

1 tsp garlic powder*

½ tsp black pepper*

1 tsp basil*

1 bay leaf *(to be removed after cooking sauce)*

½ tsp oregano*

1 package frozen chopped spinach (defrost in microwave, drain, and add to sauce when cooked)

1 package whole wheat lasagna noodles (Hodgson Mill)

12 ounces low-fat cottage cheese

8 ounces low fat shredded mozzarella cheese

1 cup grated low-fat Parmesan cheese

Note: Tastes better when prepared the day before and refrigerated—then bake.

1. In large heavy pan sauté onion. Lightly brown and drain. Add tomatoes, paste, water, parsley, salt, garlic powder, pepper, basil, bay leaf, and oregano. Simmer, uncovered, stirring occasionally, about 30 minutes, then add drained spinach.
2. Meanwhile, cook noodles as directed; drain. In large long casserole dish, alternate layers of noodles, sauce, cottage cheese, mozzarella,

(continued)

Spinach Lasagna (*continued*)

and Parmesan cheese—repeat; you will have 3 layers. DO NOT put cottage cheese on the top layer—it will burn).

3. Bake at 350°F for 40 to 50 minutes until lightly browned and bubbling. Let stand for 15 minutes; cut in squares to serve.

NUTRITION

Each serving provides:	Carbohydrates: 47 g
Calories: 343	Sugar: 7 g
Total fat: 7 g	Total fiber: 6 g
Saturated fat: 4.5 g	Protein: 23 g
Monounsaturated fat: 2 g	Iron: 2.5 mg
Polyunsaturated fat: 0.5 g	Magnesium: 81 mg
Cholesterol: 20 mg	Calcium: 401 mg
Sodium: 600 mg	Vitamin A: 2,567 IU
Potassium: 940 mg	Vitamin C: 32 mg
	Vitamin D: 0 µg

Omelet Casserole

YIELD: 8 SERVINGS

Use the egg substitute for a lower-cholesterol version and experiment with vegetables such as sliced mushrooms, bell peppers, and tomatoes for extra nutrition.

Ingredients
4 cups whole wheat bread, cubed
1½ cups shredded Swiss cheese (low sodium)
2 cups egg substitute
3 cups fat-free (skim) milk
½ teaspoon salt
¾ teaspoon Worcestershire sauce
¾ cup onion, chopped
⅛ cup diced roasted red bell pepper
⅛ cup diced green bell pepper
4 slices cooked turkey bacon, chopped
1 tablespoon chopped fresh basil*
Pepper to taste*

1. Grease 9-by-12-inch baking dish. Arrange bread cubes on the bottom of dish and sprinkle with cheese.
2. Mix together eggs, milk, salt, and Worcestershire sauce. Add onions, red and green pepper, turkey bacon, and basil to egg mixture. Pour mixture over bread and cheese. Season with pepper to taste.
3. Cover and refrigerate for 1 to 2 hours or overnight.
4. Preheat oven to 325°F. Bake 50 to 60 minutes until top is golden and eggs are set. Cut into 8 squares and serve.

NUTRITION	
Each serving provides:	Carbohydrates: 20 g
Calories: 262	Sugar: 8 g
Total fat: 10 g	Total fiber: 2.5 g
Saturated fat: 5 g	Protein: 23 g
Monounsaturated fat: 3 g	Iron: 4 mg
Polyunsaturated fat: 2 g	Magnesium: 31 mg
Cholesterol: 31 mg	Calcium: 470 mg
Sodium: 676 mg	Vitamin A: 877 IU
Potassium: 474 mg	Vitamin C: 8 mg
	Vitamin D: 1 µg

Salmon Almondine

YIELD: 2 SERVINGS

Ingredients

2 (4-ounce portions) skinless salmon fillets

2 tbsp margarine

3 tbsp sliced almonds

1½ tsp fresh squeezed lemon juice

2 tsp fresh chopped parsley

1. Preheat oven to 400°F.
2. Spray an 8-by-8-inch baking pan lightly with cooking spray. Place salmon fillets in pan and bake for 10 to 15 minutes.
3. Prepare sauce while fish fillets are baking.
4. Melt margarine in small saucepan over medium heat. Add almonds and sauté until golden brown (approximately 8 minutes). Stir frequently.
5. Remove pan from heat and add lemon juice while stirring lightly.
6. Place cooked salmon on serving plates. Pour sauce over salmon and garnish with the chopped parsley.

NUTRITION

Serving size: 1 four-ounce fish fillet	Carbohydrates: 6 g
Each serving provides:	Sugar: 1 g
Calories: 233	Total fiber: 2 g
Total fat: 13 g	Protein: 23 g
Saturated fat: 3 g	Iron: 1.3 mg
Monounsaturated fat: 7 g	Magnesium: 1.2 mg
Polyunsaturated fat: 3 g	Calcium: 46 mg
Cholesterol: 25 mg	Vitamin A: 468 IU
Sodium: 548 mg	Vitamin C: 3.5 mg
Potassium: 349 mg	Vitamin D: 1.8 µg

Lemon Tarragon Chicken

YIELD: 12 SERVINGS

Ingredients

2 tbsp margarine

8 medium skinless, boneless chicken breast halves (about 1½ pounds)

2 fresh mushrooms, halved

2 garlic cloves, minced

3 tbsp dry sherry

½ tsp dried tarragon, crushed

½ tsp lemon pepper seasoning

1¾ cups low-sodium chicken broth

⅓ cup flour

¼ cup light sour cream

Egg noodles or pasta of your choice

1. In a 12-inch skillet, melt margarine over medium heat. Add chicken, mushrooms, garlic, sherry, tarragon, and lemon pepper seasoning. Cook, uncovered, for 10 to 12 minutes or until chicken is no longer pink.
2. Remove chicken and mushrooms with slotted spoon.
3. In a screw-top jar combine chicken broth and flour and shake well until blended. Add mixture to the skillet and cook and stir over medium-high heat until mixture is thick and bubbly.
4. Remove about half of the mixture from the skillet and stir into sour cream. Return to skillet along with chicken and mushrooms. Heat through but do not boil.
5. Serve over hot cooked noodles.

NUTRITION

Each serving provides:	
Calories: 223	Carbohydrates: 32 g
Total fat: 3 g	Sugar: <1 g
Saturated fat: 1 g	Total fiber: 1.5 g
Monounsaturated fat: 1.5 g	Protein: 17 g
Polyunsaturated fat: 0.5 g	Iron: 2.5 mg
Cholesterol: 64 mg	Magnesium: 24 mg
Sodium: 426 mg	Calcium: 24 mg
Potassium: 95 mg	Vitamin A: 115 IU
	Vitamin C: 2.8 mg
	Vitamin D: 0.4 µg

Spanish Chicken and Shrimp Paella

YIELD: 8 SERVINGS

Ingredients

1 cup long-grain rice

1 pound skinless, boneless chicken breast, cut into ½-inch pieces

¼ cup olive oil

1 can (10½ oz) low-sodium chicken broth

½ pound medium-size shrimp, peeled and cleaned

½ cup frozen green peas

⅓ cup red bell pepper, chopped

⅓ cup green onion, thinly sliced

⅓ cup yellow onion, chopped

2 garlic cloves, minced

¼ tsp black pepper*

¼ tsp ground saffron

1. Cook rice and set aside.
2. Combine chicken, olive oil, and broth in a 2-quart casserole dish with a lid. Microwave on high for 4 to 5 minutes.
3. Stir in shrimp, peas, bell pepper, onions, garlic, black pepper, and saffron. Cover and microwave on high for 3½ to 4½ minutes or until shrimp turns pink.
4. Stir in cooked rice. Cover and let stand 5 minutes and then serve.

NUTRITION	
Serving size: ½ cup	Carbohydrates: 10 g
Each serving provides:	Sugar: 1.5 g
Calories: 139	Total fiber: 1 g
Total fat: 2.5 g	Protein: 19 g
Saturated fat: 0.5 g	Iron: 1.5 mg
Monounsaturated fat: 1.5 g	Magnesium: 20 mg
Polyunsaturated fat: 0.5 g	Calcium: 30 mg
Cholesterol: 70 mg	Vitamin A: 621 IU
Sodium: 400 mg	Vitamin C: 22.5 mg
Potassium: 173 mg	Vitamin D: 0 µg

Spicy Santa Fe Chicken Fajitas

Ingredients

1 pound boneless, skinless chicken breast
¼ tsp pepper*
1 clove garlic, minced
1 tsp chili powder
2 tbsp lime juice
1 tbsp fresh cilantro, chopped
1 tbsp canola oil
1 cup tomato, chopped
2 tbsp fresh cilantro, chopped
1 tbsp red onion, chopped
¼ tsp garlic, minced
10 flour tortillas (7-inch)
3 cups lettuce, shredded
½ cup light sour cream

1. Sprinkle chicken with pepper, 1 clove minced garlic, chili powder, lime juice, 1 tbsp cilantro, and oil. Turn to coat. Cover and marinate in refrigerator for 3 hours or more.
2. To make salsa, combine tomato, 2 tbsp cilantro, onion, and ¼ tsp garlic in a small bowl. Let stand 1 hour.
3. Broil chicken 6 inches from heat for 10 minutes on each side. Cut into strips. While chicken cooks, wrap tortillas in aluminum foil and warm in oven for 8 minutes.
4. To serve, wrap chicken, salsa, lettuce, and sour cream in warm tortillas.

NUTRITION	
Each serving provides:	Carbohydrates: 42 g
Calories: 286	Sugar: <1 g
Total fat: 6 g	Total fiber: 3 g
Saturated fat: 2 g	Protein: 16 g
Monounsaturated fat: 3 g	Iron: 2.9 mg
Polyunsaturated fat: 1 g	Magnesium: 24 mg
Cholesterol: 25 mg	Calcium: 50 mg
Sodium: 624 mg	Vitamin A: 120 IU
Potassium: 199 mg	Vitamin C: 7 mg
	Vitamin D: 0 µg

Asian Pork-Fried Rice

YIELD: 6 SERVINGS

Ingredients

3 tbsp canola oil

2 cloves garlic, minced

¼ cup green onion, chopped

⅔ cup carrot, chopped

½ cup cooked pork loin, chopped

4 cups cooked rice

1 tsp low-sodium soy sauce

½ cup frozen green peas

1½ cups low-cholesterol egg substitute, scrambled and chopped

¼ tsp dry mustard*

1. Heat oil in large skillet over medium heat. Add garlic and cook until soft. Stir in onion and carrot and cook for 2 minutes.
2. Add pork, rice, and soy sauce. Stir and cook for 3 minutes.
3. Add remaining ingredients and cook until thoroughly heated.

NUTRITION

Serving size: 1 cup	Carbohydrates: 39 g
Each serving provides:	Sugar: 2 g
Calories: 277	Total fiber: 1 g
Total fat: 7.2 g	Protein: 14 g
Saturated fat: 0.7 g	Iron: 3 mg
Monounsaturated fat: 4.5 g	Magnesium: 21 mg
Polyunsaturated fat: 2 g	Calcium: 32 mg
Cholesterol: 8 mg	Vitamin A: 1,816 IU
Sodium: 180 mg	Vitamin C: 4 mg
Potassium: 218 mg	Vitamin D: 1 µg

Louisiana-Style Shrimp Creole

Ingredients

1 pound fresh or frozen medium shrimp in shells
¾ cup chopped onion
1 stalk chopped celery
¾ cup green bell pepper, chopped
2 cloves garlic
2 tbsp canola oil
1 can (14.5 oz) diced tomatoes (low sodium), undrained
¼ tsp cayenne pepper
⅛ tsp salt
½ tsp paprika*
1 tbsp fresh parsley
2 cups cooked rice

1. Peel and devein shrimp, removing tails. Rinse and pat dry; set aside.
2. In a large skillet, cook onion, celery, bell pepper, and garlic in hot oil over medium heat for ~5 minutes or until tender. Stir in undrained tomatoes, cayenne pepper, salt, and paprika. Bring to a boil, then reduce heat and simmer, uncovered, for 5 to 8 minutes or until thickened.
3. Stir shrimp and parsley into the mixture. Stir frequently for 2 to 4 minutes or until shrimp is done. Serve over rice.

NUTRITION

Each serving provides:	
Calories: 259	Carbohydrates: 31 g
Total fat: 7 g	Sugar: 6 g
Saturated fat: 0.4 g	Total fiber: 2.5 g
Monounsaturated fat: 4 g	Protein: 18 g
Polyunsaturated fat: 2.5 g	Iron: 4 mg
Cholesterol: 134 mg	Magnesium: 52 mg
Sodium: 212 mg	Calcium: 82 mg
Potassium: 555 mg	Vitamin A: 214 IU
	Vitamin C: 47 mg
	Vitamin D: 2.5 µg

Seared Garlic Scallops

Ingredients

1 pound fresh or frozen sea scallops

3 cloves garlic, minced

1 tbsp butter

2 tbsp dry white wine

1 tbsp fresh chives

1. Thaw scallops if frozen. Rinse scallops and pat dry.
2. In a skillet, cook garlic in ½ tbsp hot butter over medium-high heat for 30 seconds. Add scallops.
3. Cook, stirring frequently, for 2 to 4 minutes or until scallops turn opaque. Remove from skillet and transfer to a serving platter.
4. Add the remaining ½ tbsp butter and wine to the skillet. Cook and stir to loosen any browned bits. Pour over scallops; sprinkle with chives.

NUTRITION	
Each serving provides:	Carbohydrates: 3.5 g
Calories: 138	Sugar: 0 g
Total fat: 5.5 g	Total fiber: 0 g
Saturated fat: 2.5 g	Protein: 18.5 g
Monounsaturated fat: 2 g	Iron: 0.4 mg
Polyunsaturated fat: 1 g	Magnesium: 62 mg
Cholesterol: 44 mg	Calcium: 34 mg
Sodium: 539 mg	Vitamin A: 79 IU
Potassium: 339 mg	Vitamin C: 4 mg
	Vitamin D: 0.1 µg

Vegetable-Flounder Bake

Ingredients

1 pound flounder fillets
(~¾ inch thick)
2 cups carrots, sliced thin,
  lightly cooked
2 cups fresh mushroom, sliced
½ zucchini, sliced
½ cup green onion, chopped

2 tsp lemon zest*
½ tsp dried oregano*
⅛ tsp salt
¼ tsp black pepper*
4 cloves garlic, halved
2 tsp olive oil
2 medium oranges, sliced thin

1. Thaw fish if frozen. Rinse fish and pat dry. Cut into 4 pieces.
2. Cut four 24-inch pieces of wide aluminum foil. Fold each in half to make four 18-by-12-inch pieces.
3. In a large bowl, combine carrots, mushrooms, zucchini, green onion, lemon zest, oregano, salt, pepper, and garlic.
4. Divide vegetables into 4 pieces of foil, placing the vegetables in the center of the foil. Place one flounder fillet piece on top of each vegetable portion.
5. Drizzle ½ tsp olive oil over each flounder piece. Top with orange slices and seal foil together with a double fold. Be sure to completely enclose all edges of foil, allowing space for steam to build. Place the foiled flounder-vegetable bake on a baking pan.
6. Bake at 350°F for ~20 to 30 minutes or until fish begins to flake with a fork. Open foil carefully to allow steam to escape.

NUTRITION

Each serving provides:

Calories: 239	Carbohydrates: 18 g
Total fat: 7 g	Sugar: 12 g
Saturated fat: 1 g	Total fiber: 4 g
Monounsaturated fat: 4 g	Protein: 26 g
Polyunsaturated fat: 2 g	Iron: 1.1 mg
Cholesterol: 49 mg	Calcium: 80 mg
Sodium: 305 mg	Vitamin A: 0 IU
Potassium: 217 mg	Vitamin C: 4.8 mg
	Vitamin D: 0 µg

Caribbean Orange Roughy

Ingredients

1½ pounds orange roughy
¼ cup fresh cilantro
1 tsp lime zest
1¼ tbsp lime juice
1 tbsp butter, melted
Black pepper to taste*

1. Cut fish into 4 serving-size pieces.
2. Place fish onto a greased broiler pan. Broil until fish begins to flake. (Allow 4 to 6 minutes per ½-inch thickness of fish.)
3. Meanwhile, in a small bowl combine cilantro, lime zest, lime juice, melted butter.
4. Spoon cilantro mix over fish and serve.

NUTRITION

Each serving provides:	
Calories: 156	Carbohydrates: 2 g
Total fat: 4 g	Sugar: 0 g
Saturated fat: 2 g	Total fiber: 0 g
Monounsaturated fat: 2 g	Protein: 28 g
Polyunsaturated fat: 0 g	Iron: 1.2 mg
Cholesterol: 42 mg	Magnesium: 18 mg
Sodium: 258 mg	Calcium: 50 mg
Potassium: 175 mg	Vitamin A: 0 IU
	Vitamin C: 3 mg
	Vitamin D: 0 µg

[116]   **Bringing Down High Blood Pressure**

Herb-Marinated Lamb Chops

Ingredients

4 lamb loin chops (lean)

¼ cup olive oil

2 tbsp lemon juice

2 tsp lemon zest*

2 garlic cloves, minced

½ tsp dried basil*

½ tsp dried rosemary, crushed

½ tsp black pepper*

1. Trim fat from lamb chops.
2. Combine remaining ingredients in a resealable plastic bag. Place lamp chops in bag and seal. Turn to coat thoroughly; refrigerate overnight.
3. Drain and discard marinade. Broil lamb 3 to 4 inches from heat for 4 to 6 minutes on each side or until meat reaches desired doneness.

NUTRITION

Each serving provides:	
Calories: 181	Carbohydrates: 1 g
Total fat: 15 g	Sugar: 0 g
Saturated fat: 3 g	Total fiber: 0 g
Monounsaturated fat: 11 g	Protein: 10.5 g
Polyunsaturated fat: 1 g	Iron: 1 mg
Cholesterol: 32 mg	Magnesium: 11 mg
Sodium: 29 mg	Calcium: 15 mg
Potassium: 154 mg	Vitamin A: 2 IU
	Vitamin C: 4 mg
	Vitamin D: 0.1 µg

Vegetable Orzo Primavera

Ingredients

1 tbsp olive oil

1 cup uncooked orzo pasta

1 clove garlic, crushed

1 medium zucchini, shredded

1 medium carrot, shredded

1 can (14 oz) low-sodium vegetable broth

1 lemon, zested (or zest of 1 lemon)*

1 tbsp fresh thyme, chopped

¼ cup grated Parmesan cheese

1. Heat the oil in a pot over medium heat. Stir in orzo, and cook 2 minutes, until golden.
2. Stir in garlic, zucchini, and carrot, and cook another 2 minutes.
3. Pour in the broth and mix in lemon zest. Bring to a boil. Reduce heat to low and simmer for 10 minutes, or until liquid has been absorbed and orzo is tender.
4. Season with thyme and top with Parmesan to serve.

NUTRITION

Each serving provides:

Calories: 123	Carbohydrates: 14 g
Total fat: 5 g	Sugar: 1 g
Saturated fat: 1.5 g	Total fiber: 1.2 g
Monounsaturated fat: 3 g	Protein: 5.5 g
Polyunsaturated fat: 0.5 g	Iron: 0.5 mg
Cholesterol: 5 mg	Magnesium: 13 mg
Sodium: 561 mg	Calcium: 95 mg
Potassium: 97 mg	Vitamin A: 528 IU
	Vitamin C: 3 mg
	Vitamin D: 0 µg

Almond-Crusted Tilapia

Ingredients

2 eggs

1 tsp lemon pepper

1 tsp garlic pepper

1 cup almonds, ground

1 cup freshly grated Parmesan cheese

8 (6-ounce) tilapia fillets

¼ cup all-purpose flour for dusting

½ cup freshly grated Parmesan cheese

8 sprigs parsley

8 lemon wedges

1. Beat the eggs with the lemon pepper and garlic pepper until blended; set aside. Stir together ground almonds with 1 cup of Parmesan cheese in a shallow dish until combined; set aside. Dust the tilapia fillets with flour, and shake off excess. Dip the tilapia in egg, then press into the almond mixture.

2. In a large skillet over medium-high heat, cook tilapia in cooking spray until golden brown on both sides, 2 to 3 minutes per side. Reduce heat to medium. Sprinkle the tilapia with the remaining ½ cup of Parmesan cheese, cover, and continue cooking until the Parmesan cheese has melted, about 5 minutes.

3. Transfer the tilapia to a serving dish, and garnish with parsley springs and lemon wedges to serve.

NUTRITION

Each serving provides:

Calories: 280

Total fat: 12 g

  Saturated fat: 3.5 g

  Monounsaturated fat: 6 g

  Polyunsaturated fat: 2.5 g

Cholesterol: 137 mg

Sodium: 365 mg

Potassium: 512 mg

Carbohydrates: 7 g

Sugar: 0 g

Total fiber: 1.5 g

Protein: 36 g

Iron: 1 mg

Magnesium: 108 mg

Calcium: 233 mg

Vitamin A: 58 IU

Vitamin C: 4 mg

Vitamin D: 2 µg

Sautéed Calamari

Ingredients
3 garlic cloves
1¼ tbsp olive oil
2 pounds calamari
1 tsp red pepper flakes*
1 tsp flour
½ cup white wine
Freshly chopped parsley for garnish

1. Sauté garlic cloves in olive oil until golden in color and then remove the cloves. The garlic will have penetrated and flavored the oil.
2. Add the calamari, red pepper flakes, and flour. Then add the wine, simmer on low-heat, and cover for approximately 45 minutes.

NUTRITION	
Each serving provides:	Carbohydrates: 7 g
Calories: 109	Sugar: 0 g
Total fat: 3 g	Total fiber: <1 g
Saturated fat: <1 g	Protein: 13.5 g
Monounsaturated fat: 1.25 g	Iron: 1 mg
Polyunsaturated fat: 1.5 g	Magnesium: 30 mg
Cholesterol: 196 mg	Calcium: 35 mg
Sodium: 187 mg	Vitamin A: 24 IU
Potassium: 340 mg	Vitamin C: 5 mg
	Vitamin D: <1 µg

MARINADES, SEASONINGS, AND RUBS

Dried spices such as cayenne pepper flakes, thyme, cumin, nutmeg, allspice, and rubbed sage are ideal for creating marinades and rubs for fish, poultry, lamb, pork and beef, as you'll see in the following recipes.

The marinades and rubs in this section take the guesswork out of cooking with flavor. You can opt for these recipes, or you can experiment with condiments to jazz up your food:

Condiments

- Honey mustard, Dijonnaise mustard, low-carb ketchup, and light mayonnaise
- Jam, jelly, or honey. If you have diabetes, try low-sugar varieties.
- Salsa made from fresh produce.
- Use Splenda sweetener or stevia instead of sugar, especially if you have diabetes.
- Fresh lemon or lime juice.
- Store-brand cooking sprays made with olive oil and other unsaturated fat oils.
- Vinegars: balsamic, apple cider, sherry, champagne, white and red wine, and tarragon.
- Prepared horseradish.
- If you use soy sauce, chipotle sauce, or Worcestershire sauce, use only the low-sodium varieties or use sparingly.
- Sweet pickle relish.

Fresh herbs like oregano, basil, rosemary, tarragon, and Italian flat-leaf parsley are now available in the produce section of many grocery stores. Cut fresh herbs sell for between $2.99 and $4.00, depending on where you shop. Tiny whole plants sell for around the same price or less and will provide an ongoing supply if watered and nurtured in a sunny kitchen window or patio container.

Look for Dr. Rhoden's FlavorDoctor for healthy salt-free grilling and seasoning combinations.

Island-Style Grilling Marinade

YIELD: 24 SERVINGS

Ingredients

6 cloves garlic, coarsely chopped

½ cup minced yellow onion

1 cup freshly squeezed orange juice

½ cup freshly squeezed lime juice

½ tsp ground cumin*

1 tsp dried oregano flakes*

½ tsp lemon-pepper seasoning

½ tsp freshly ground black pepper*

1 tsp kosher salt

¼ cup chopped cilantro

1 tsp hot pepper sauce (e.g., Tabasco™) (optional)

1 cup olive oil

1. Pulse the garlic and onion in a blender until very finely chopped. Pour in orange juice and lime juice; season with cumin, oregano, lemon pepper, black pepper, salt, cilantro, and hot pepper sauce. Blend until thoroughly incorporated. Pour in the olive oil, and blend until smooth.

Note: Meat and chicken should be marinated overnight and fish only needs 1 hour to marinate.

NUTRITION	
Serving size: 2 tbsp	Carbohydrates: 2 g
Each serving provides:	Sugar: 0 g
Calories: 86	Total fiber: 0 g
Total fat: 8.5 g	Protein: 0.2 g
Saturated fat: 1.2 g	Iron: <1 mg
Monounsaturated fat: 6.5 g	Magnesium: 2.5 mg
Polyunsaturated fat: 0.8 g	Calcium: 5 mg
Cholesterol: 0 mg	Vitamin A: 3.9 IU
Sodium: 50 mg	Vitamin C: 7 mg
Potassium: 103 mg	Vitamin D: 0 µg

Fabulous Fajita Marinade

YIELD: 8 SERVINGS

Ingredients

¼ cup beer

⅓ cup fresh lime juice

1 tbsp olive oil

2 cloves garlic, minced

1 tbsp brown sugar

1 tbsp Worcestershire sauce

1 tbsp chopped cilantro

½ tsp ground cumin*

Salt, to taste

1. To prepare the marinade, stir together beer, lime juice, olive oil, garlic, brown sugar, Worcestershire sauce, cilantro, cumin, and salt; mix well.

2. To use marinade, pour into a resealable plastic bag, add up to 1½ pounds of chicken breast, and mix until chicken is well coated. Marinate for at least 1 to 3 hours in the refrigerator.

NUTRITION	
Serving size: 2 tbsp	Carbohydrates: 3 g
Each serving provides:	Sugar: 0 g
Calories: 30	Total fiber: 0 g
Total fat: 1.5 g	Protein: <1 g
Saturated fat: 0.2 g	Iron: <1 mg
Monounsaturated fat: 1.2 g	Magnesium: 3 mg
Polyunsaturated fat: 0.1 g	Calcium: 4.5 mg
Cholesterol: 0 mg	Vitamin A: 0.5 IU
Sodium: 58 mg	Vitamin C: 3.2 mg
Potassium: 26 mg	Vitamin D: 0 µg

Cajun Spice Rub

Ingredients

2 tbsp paprika*

1 tbsp cumin, ground*

1 tbsp dried thyme

4 garlic cloves, minced

1 onion, diced

1 tbsp dried oregano*

1 tsp black pepper*

1 tsp cayenne pepper

1. Combine all ingredients and thoroughly rub on meat. Allow meat to marinate for at least 2 hours prior to cooking.

NUTRITION

Each serving provides:	
Calories: 45	Carbohydrates: 8 g
Total fat: 0.75 g	Sugar: <1 g
Saturated fat: <1 g	Total fiber: 2.5 g
Monounsaturated fat: <1 g	Protein: 1.5 g
Polyunsaturated fat: 0.5 g	Iron: 2 mg
Cholesterol: 0 mg	Magnesium: 20 mg
Sodium: 3.5 mg	Calcium: 64 mg
Potassium: 228 mg	Vitamin A: 245 IU
	Vitamin C: 7.5 mg
	Vitamin D: 0 µg

DESSERTS

Brandy Apple Crisp

YIELD: 6 SERVINGS

Ingredients

4 cups tart apples, peeled and chopped

3 tbsp sugar

3 tbsp brandy

2 tsp lemon juice

½ tsp cinnamon

⅛ tsp nutmeg

¾ cup dry oats

¼ cup brown sugar

2 tbsp flour

2 tbsp margarine

1. Combine first 6 ingredients in an 8-inch square baking pan. Toss well; set aside.
2. Combine oats, brown sugar, and flour in a small bowl. Cut in margarine until well-blended. Sprinkle over apple mixture.
3. Bake at 350°F for 45 minutes.

NUTRITION	
Serving size: ½ cup	Carbohydrates: 40 g
Each serving provides:	Sugar: 15 g
Calories: 184	Total fiber: 4 g
Total fat: 2 g	Protein: 1.3 g
Saturated fat: 0.5 g	Iron: 0.8 mg
Monounsaturated fat: 0.5 g	Magnesium: 17 mg
Polyunsaturated fat: 1 g	Calcium: 22 mg
Cholesterol: 0 mg	Vitamin A: 24 IU
Sodium: 28 mg	Vitamin C: 8.8 mg
Potassium: 202 mg	Vitamin D: 0 µg

Green Tea Cakes

Note: The tea called for here is matcha, a powdered green tea used in the Japanese tea ceremony. It is unnecessary to buy the highest-grade tea for this recipe.

YIELD: 12 SERVINGS

Ingredients

4 eggs + 1 egg yolk, divided

½ cup sugar

⅓ cup cake flour

2 tbsp cornstarch

2 tbsp powdered green tea

⅛ tsp cream of tartar

2 tbsp confectioners' sugar

6 tbsp almond paste

1 cup heavy cream

4 tsp superfine sugar

1. Preheat oven to 450°F.
2. With an electric mixer, beat 2 whole eggs, 3 egg yolks, and 7 tablespoons sugar together until thick and tripled in volume, about 5 minutes.
3. Sift together flour, cornstarch, and 1 tablespoon green tea. Sift mixture onto beaten eggs and fold in. Beat egg whites with cream of tartar until soft peaks form. Beat in remaining 1 tablespoon sugar until stiff. Fold into batter. Spread batter in a shallow 11-by-7-inch pan that has been greased and lined with greased and floured wax paper.
4. Bake until lightly browned and springy to touch. Loosen edges of cake. Sprinkle with confectioners' sugar, then cover with a kitchen towel and invert onto a flat surface. Let cool. Using a biscuit cutter or other decorative cutter, cut out 24 pieces of cake.
5. Knead almond paste with 1 teaspoon green tea. Roll out thinly between sheets of plastic wrap. Using a small cookie cutter, cut out 12 decorative shapes.

6. Gradually whisk heavy cream into superfine sugar and remaining 2 teaspoons green tea, then beat until not quite stiff. To assemble cakes, sandwich two cake layers with about ¼ inch green tea whipped cream. Frost top and sides with whipped cream and decorate with almond paste cutouts. Chill until serving.

Modified and reprinted with permission from GourMAsia.

NUTRITION

Serving size: 1 petit four	Carbohydrates: 17 g
Each serving provides:	Sugar: 6 g
Calories: 197	Total fiber: 0.5 g
Total fat: 12.5 g	Protein: 4 g
Saturated fat: 5.5 g	Iron: 0.5 mg
Monounsaturated fat: 5.5 g	Magnesium: 28 mg
Polyunsaturated fat: 1.5 g	Calcium: 43 mg
Cholesterol: 98 mg	Vitamin A: 115 IU
Sodium: 30 mg	Vitamin C: <1 mg
Potassium: 100 mg	Vitamin D: 0.5 µg

Maple Crisp Bars

Ingredients

⅓ cup margarine

1 cup sugar

1 tsp maple extract

½ cup maple pancake syrup (not pure maple syrup)

8 cups puffed rice cereal

1. In a large saucepan, melt margarine over medium heat. Stir in sugar, extract, and syrup; bring to a boil. Remove from heat.
2. Stir in cereal, coating it well the with the sugar mixture.
3. Press into a greased 13-by-9-inch baking pan. Chill. Cut into 20 bars.

NUTRITION

Each serving provides:	
Calories: 156	Carbohydrates: 34 g
Total fat: 2 g	Sugar: 10 g
Saturated fat: 0.5 g	Total fiber: <1 g
Monounsaturated fat: 0.5 g	Protein: 0.5 g
Polyunsaturated fat: 1 g	Iron: 0.5 mg
Cholesterol: 0 mg	Magnesium: 4.5 mg
Sodium: 33 mg	Calcium: 10 mg
Potassium: 40 mg	Vitamin A: 22.5 IU
	Vitamin C: 0 mg
	Vitamin D: 0 µg

Tasty Rice Pudding

Ingredients

3 cups low-fat milk

⅓ cup uncooked rice

⅓ cup raisins (or dried fruit of your choice)

¼ cup sugar

1 tsp vanilla

¼ tsp ground nutmeg

⅛ tsp cinnamon

1. In a medium saucepan, bring milk just to boiling. Stir in uncooked rice and raisins. Cook, covered, over low heat for approximately 30 minutes or until most of the milk is absorbed, stirring occasionally. (Mixture may appear curdled.)
2. Remove saucepan from heat. Stir in sugar and vanilla.
3. Mix nutmeg and cinnamon together in a separate bowl and sprinkle on top of pudding just before serving. Serve warm or chilled.

NUTRITION

Each serving provides:	
Calories: 150	Carbohydrates: 29 g
Total fat: 1.5 g	Sugar: 10 g
Saturated fat: 0.8 g	Total fiber: 0.5 g
Monounsaturated fat: 0.4 g	Protein: 5 g
Polyunsaturated fat: <0.5 g	Iron: 0.8 mg
Cholesterol: 5 mg	Magnesium: 22 mg
Sodium: 63 mg	Calcium: 159 mg
Potassium: 264 mg	Vitamin A: 72 IU
	Vitamin C: 1.5 mg
	Vitamin D: 1 µg

Refreshing Orange-Pineapple Sherbet

YIELD: 10 SERVINGS

Ingredients

1½ cups orange juice

1 cup sugar

3 cups milk, scalded and cooled

1 can (15 oz) crushed pineapple (in its own juice)

1 tsp grated orange peel

1. In a bowl, combine orange juice and sugar; blend thoroughly. Add milk and mix.
2. Place in a chilled shallow pan (9 × 13 inches). Freeze until mushy. Then place mushy mixture in a mixing bowl and whip. Add pineapple and grated orange peel. Return to shallow pan and freeze.

NUTRITION

Each serving provides:	
Calories: 155	Carbohydrates: 34 g
Total fat: 1 g	Sugar: 12 g
Saturated fat: 0.5 g	Total fiber: 0.4 g
Monounsaturated fat: 0.2 g	Protein: 2.5 g
Polyunsaturated fat: <0.1 g	Iron: <1 mg
Cholesterol: 3 mg	Magnesium: 20 mg
Sodium: 38 mg	Calcium: 100 mg
Potassium: 241 mg	Vitamin A: 53 IU
	Vitamin C: 23 mg
	Vitamin D: 0.7 µg

Chapter 5

EXERCISING TO SAVE YOUR LIFE

WE'VE ALL HEARD the catchphrases: "Feel the burn. Get your body moving. No pain, no gain." The fitness experts who promote their own fitness products, Web sites, DVDs, TV shows, and books might as well say, "No pain, lots of weight gain, heart problems, high blood pressure, and shortened life span." One of my favorite cartoons is from Randy Glasbergen (2003)—a doctor asks his patient, "What fits your busy schedule better, exercising one hour a day or being dead 24 hours a day??"

This perfectly sums up the truth about exercise. Did you know that complications of diabetes and other diseases of the heart and arteries can be very painful and debilitating over time? As many as 12 percent of all deaths in the United States, 250,000 per year, may be attributed indirectly to lack of regular physical activity. This fact has been well publicized over the years, but amazingly enough, only about one in four Americans exercises enough to be considered physically active. Overall, our nation does not meet physical activity requirements. A recent survey by the Centers for Disease Control found that more than 22 percent of Americans did not engage in any physical activity within a month! This statistic, perhaps not coincidentally, topped 30 percent in those states with the highest rates of obesity.

Some people may argue that exercise is overrated, that genetics determine our health. Genetics do play a role, but if you look at all the famous examples of celebrities that seem to be blessed with natural beauty but have been lampooned by the press for being out of shape, you realize that genetics are no guarantee of future fitness. Genetic factors don't excuse us from exercising. Regular exercise can protect you from the effects of genetic predisposition to heart disease, although genetics influence specific responses of blood pressure to exercise training. For most of us, they are also not excuses for being inactive, as there are few conditions that make it impossible to exercise. However, some may have more challenges than others. If you fit in this category, you may benefit from the later section in this chapter titled "Help for the Exercise-Challenged." A common question people ask me as a specialist in exercise physiology is, "How do I exercise if my physical condition makes it difficult?"

Whenever I speak to groups, another frequent question is, "Could you recommend the best exercise book?" I tell people that there are several good exercise books out there, but reading one won't make you fit. What people really mean is, "Help me. Show me how. Get me started. I don't have a lot of time to achieve the results I need and want. I don't even know if I'm worth the investment."

I want to say to you right now that you are worth the time and energy exercise takes! You are worth the investment needed to bring down your blood pressure below 120/80. You bought this book, or as so often happens, someone gave it to you because someone thinks you are worth the effort. Someone you love, a friend or family member, or perhaps someone whose job it is to care about your health, such as your doctor, sees the exercise deficit in your life. That person may already know the importance of exercise as a healthy lifestyle, and may possess the rest of the pieces of the overall picture that you don't currently have. That person is trying to give you a greater gift, as I am. And once you accept that gift, once you get hooked on exercise, hopefully there's no going back. My goal in this chapter is to inspire you to make fitness a way of life!

The Gift of Motion

We talked in Chapter 3 about the way that the body burns fuel when we're active and stores fuel when we're sedentary. You can ask why anyone would want to sit all day with excess fuel that just clings to you and needs to move around, to burn, and to dance. Many people who sit around all day have forgotten how great exercise feels. Exercise doesn't have to be your favorite thing or what you love to do most, but you can recapture the joy and pleasure you once took in it. Yes, I said pleasure. You may think of exercise as a chore and a burden, especially if you're out of shape, but it's far preferable than the alternative of poor health.

And even if you associate exercise only with memories of junior high locker rooms, gym class, dodgeball, and getting teased by your peers (as well as the coach), physical fitness can be highly enjoyable for adults. In fact tedious household chores—such as mowing the lawn or cleaning closets—can even be more favorable when the benefits of staying active are understood. My goal is to inspire you to get active.

To make the exercise investment, and more importantly, to enjoy exercise, it is important to have the right mind-set. Hopefully, Chapter 2 was a prompt to get moving and choose healthy habits!

Here's a sample exercise you can try. First, set the book down at eye level if you need to refer to it. Stand upright. Raise your left arm over your head. Slowly and gently, bend as far as you can to your right. Pretend you are trying to touch the opposite wall. Inhale for five seconds. Exhale and sweep your arm back down. Repeat with the right arm and reach toward the opposite wall.

That may not seem as if you've just done anything. After all, your image of fitness is people who jog at 5 a.m.! However, you have just addressed your flexibility, which is certainly an important component of overall fitness. On the other hand, for those of you who think, "Okay, I've exercised, now I'm automatically healthy," be prepared for a mental adjustment. You can't just expect one small stretching exercise to work wonders overnight if you've spent years avoiding exercise. That said, if you just did the exercise in the example, you've shown you're willing to make the time and take the time for exercise.

Those of you who like to walk and are ambulatory might try this well-known beginners' fit walking program (see Table 5.1) that many physicians have passed along to their patients.

If you have difficulty committing to a walking program, I'd like to help you "Commit to Walk," to imitate a popular smoking-cessation program. Here are my motivational suggestions:

- Ask other people to walk with you. Find a partner or a group. When you know someone else is waiting for you, it keeps you going.
- Wear comfortable shoes and good socks to help cushion your feet.
- Wear clothes that are right for the season. Try using layers of clothing in the cold weather to keep you warm, and cotton clothes in the summer to keep you cool.

Table 5.1. Beginners' Fit Walking Program

	Warm Up	Activity	Cool Down	Total Time
WEEK 1				
Session A	Walk slowly 5 min.	Then walk briskly 5 min.	Then walk slowly 5 min.	15 min.
Session B	Repeat above pattern			
Session C	Repeat above pattern			
Continue with at least three walking sessions during each week of the program.				
WEEK 2	Walk slowly 5 min.	Then walk briskly 7 min.	Then walk slowly 5 min.	17 min.
WEEK 3	Walk slowly 5 min.	Then walk briskly 9 min.	Then walk slowly 5 min.	19 min.
WEEK 4	Walk slowly 5 min.	Then walk briskly 11 min.	Then walk slowly 5 min.	21 min.
WEEK 5	Walk slowly 5 min.	Then walk briskly 13 min.	Then walk slowly 5 min.	23 min.
WEEK 6	Walk slowly 5 min.	Then walk briskly 15 min.	Then walk slowly 5 min.	25 min.
WEEK 7	Walk slowly 5 min.	Then walk briskly 18 min.	Then walk slowly 5 min.	28 min.
	Warm Up	**Activity**	**Cool Down**	**Total Time**
WEEK 8	Walk slowly 5 min.	Then walk briskly 20 min.	Then walk slowly 5 min.	30 min.
WEEK 9	Walk slowly 5 min.	Then walk briskly 23 min.	Then walk slowly 5 min.	33 min.
WEEK 10	Walk slowly 5 min.	Then walk briskly 26 min.	Then walk slowly 5 min.	36 min.
WEEK 11	Walk slowly 5 min.	Then walk briskly 28 min.	Then walk slowly 5 min.	38 min.
WEEK 12 AND BEYOND	Walk slowly 5 min.	Then walk briskly 30 min.	Then walk slowly 5 min.	40 min.

- Drink plenty of water. It doesn't have to be that fancy bottled stuff—get your own container and keep it filled with plenty of regular water. Carry it with you if you can.
- Don't forget to stretch before you walk. Try to start off slowly.
- Be safe—pay attention to your surroundings.
- Walk in a safe place that has plenty of lights in the evening. Try walking around a local school's parking lot, or going to the mall.
- Try to walk five times a week. It may seem like a lot at first, but you will gradually build up. For example, three times per week is certainly better than none!
- Try to think of your walk in three parts. Imagine a warm-up period at the beginning, challenge yourself with a brisk pace in the middle, and finally picture a cool-down. You can feel success when you finish each part.

If you do take the time for exercise, centuries of medical factual information show that you will get results.

Time *Is* on Your Side

Remember from Chapter 2 that all healthy adults aged 18 to 65 should aim for moderate-intensity (preferably aerobic) physical activity for a minimum of 30 minutes 5 days a week. Being physically active is one of the most important things you can do to prevent or control high blood pressure. It also helps to reduce your risk of heart disease. We gave the example of walking one mile a day. That example shows that it doesn't require a lot of effort to become physically active. All you need is 30 minutes of moderate-level physical activity on most days of the week. And don't forget that physical activity adds up (i.e., 10 minutes here, 10 minutes there) as we will see shortly.

What do we mean when we say moderate? Think of your most intensive, hardest bouts of physical activity—vigorous hiking, an hour of dancing at a rock concert, rock climbing, hauling boxes up a flight of stairs. Decrease that intensity to about 70 to 85 percent of your hardest physical effort. Examples include brisk walking, bicycling, raking leaves, and gardening. Table 5.2 gives suggestions to get you started.

You'll notice that in this table, we included activities that are performed longer than 30 minutes, or even actions such as shoveling snow that you do for a 15-minute stretch. You can divide the 30 minutes

Table 5.2. Exercise Activities

Common Activities	Sporting Activities
■ Washing and waxing a car for 45–60 minutes	■ Playing volleyball for 45–60 minutes
■ Washing windows or floors for 45–60 minutes	■ Playing touch football for 45 minutes
■ Gardening for 30–45 minutes	■ Walking 2 miles in 30 minutes (1 mile in 15 minutes)
■ Wheeling self in wheelchair for 30–40 minutes	■ Dancing fast (social) for 30 minutes
■ Pushing a stroller 1½ miles in 30 minutes	■ Jumping rope for 15 minutes
■ Raking leaves for 30 minutes	■ Rebounding or jumping on a trampoline for 10–20 minutes
■ Shoveling snow for 15 minutes	■ Doing gentle yoga for 10–15 minutes, or doing a 10-minute quick stretch-and-flex workout
■ Stair walking for 15 minutes	
■ Walking from a bus stop two stops before your destination for 10 minutes	■ Exercising on a manual stairstepper for 10 minutes
■ Playing with children for 10–15 minutes	■ Horseback riding for 30 minutes
■ Walking dog for 10 minutes	■ Ice skating, roller skating, or Rollerblading for 30 minutes
■ Mowing/weeding the lawn for 10 minutes	■ Canoeing for 30 minutes
■ Pushing a shopping cart for 30 minutes	■ Golfing for 15–30 minutes
	■ Playing 30 minutes of baseball
	■ Playing 30 minutes of badminton or doubles tennis
	■ Exercising on a treadmill or stationary bike for 10 minutes

into shorter periods of at least 10 minutes each. When you work up to over 30 minutes, you can divide washing and waxing a car into two 30-minute stretches, or three intervals of 15 minutes.

Not to run this point into the ground, but you can get started by doing 30 minutes of a moderate-level activity on most, and preferably all, days of the week. Brisk walking, bicycling, and gardening are examples. If you already engage in 30 minutes of moderate-level physical activity a day, you can get added benefits by doing more. Engage a moderate-level activity for a longer period each day or engage in a more vigorous activity. One study found that nine weekly 10-minute sessions offer the same cardiovascular benefits as three weekly 30-minute sessions. That's good news for beginning exercisers, who may find it easier to stick to shorter, more manageable workouts.

In Chapter 2, we suggested walking during your lunch hour or coffee break. That coffee will taste better after an exercise break. In fact, you'll feel more alert and motivated. Try 10 minutes of brisk walking before work or school and 10 minutes of stair climbing or a quick run at noon. To prevent that after-dinner crash when you feel sleepy and have difficulty concentrating, try 10 minutes of jumping rope or cycling in the evening. You can even jump rope while you watch television if you're so inclined, without being so absorbed in the program that you take a fall! I speak from experience. Television can be an excellent creative aid to fitness, as you'll find out in a bit.

The writing group of the American College of Sports Medicine and the American Heart Association (ACSM and AHA, respectively), the recognized authorities on the effects of exercise, gives you the green light to substitute a minimum of 20 minutes of vigorous-intensity aerobic activity three days a week. Table 5.3 provides suggestions.

The difference between moderate- and vigorous-intensity activities is the increased heart rate. You'll experience a higher heart rate

Table 5.3. Vigorous-Intensity Aerobic Activities

Common Activities	*Sporting Activities*
■ Digging for 20 minutes	■ Swimming laps or doing water aerobics for 20 minutes
■ Hammering and sawing (carpentry) for 20 minutes	■ Shooting baskets (basketball) for 30 minutes
■ Carrying and hauling boxes up stairs for 20 minutes	■ Playing basketball for 15–20 minutes
■ Building brick walls (masonry) for 20 minutes	■ Playing soccer for 20 minutes
■ Heavy lifting for 20 minutes	■ Running 1½ miles in 15 minutes (1 mile in 10 minutes)
■ Vigorous rough-and-tumble play with children for 20 minutes (or more)	■ Playing racquetball or singles tennis for 10–20 minutes
■ Mopping and washing the floor for 30 minutes	■ Playing hockey for 20 minutes
	■ Doing martial arts for 20 minutes

when you do martial arts for 20 minutes than when you perform yoga or walking workouts.

Please ask your doctor before commencing this type of exercise, as it may not be suitable for everyone.

Combining exercises is also acceptable. You can meet your activity recommendations by walking briskly or by performing another activity that noticeably accelerates the heart rate for 30 minutes twice during the week and then jogging for 20 minutes, or performing any activity that causes rapid breathing and a substantial increase in heart rate on two other days. The updated ACSM/AHA guidelines specify that moderate- and vigorous-intensity exercises are complementary to daily living and that even more exercise than the recommended amount provides additional health benefits. Muscle-strengthening activities have also been included in the updated recommendations. The ACSM/AHA writing group also states that short bouts of activity—10 minutes or more—can be combined to meet the 30-minute daily goal. This additive concept is simple, since 1 + 1 always equals 2.

Use the suggestions in Table 5.2 and Table 5.3 to help you work up to your fitness goal. You can help yourself by making a list of physical activities that you enjoy. Try to include both of the following on different days:

1. Cardiovascular, also known as aerobic exercise, including walking, running, biking, swimming, dancing, or jumping rope
2. Muscle-strengthening activities such as lifting light weights or doing push-ups

Include a variety of activities to avoid boredom, and use different muscle groups. We have so many tools to help us exercise, MP3 players, iPods, TVs at home and in the gym, radios, and so on. For those who love video games, Wii Fit may be an option. Be creative and make exercise fun. If you mainly exercise on machines, as I do, you'll find plenty of safety and stability while working all your muscle groups through resistance.

What about popular exercises such as Pilates? Research on the effectiveness of the method developed by Joseph Pilates as well as the innumerable variations offered in workout videos is limited. However, most exercise science specialists agree that it is certainly beneficial for the "core" muscles, which include the abdominals and spine stability muscles. In fact, the method of Pilates is based on stabilization of the spine during the execution of all exercises while promoting conscious involvement of the deep abdominal muscles as well as controlled, smooth breathing. All this is to say that Pilates may be beneficial to improve motor control, range of motion, body composition, and injury rehabilitation. You can take a Pilates class if you think that exercising in a group will motivate you, but if you're self-conscious about your fitness level, there are plenty of Pilates routines you can do at home.

If you feel like a one-man or one-woman band, if you enjoy your "me" time but are getting restless, make exercise a shared pleasure. Go out and hit tennis balls with your spouse or walk around the neighborhood or in the park. Being active together can certainly be an inexpensive and invigorating date. Play sports with friends in an amateur, church, or community league—just keep the competition friendly and don't be overly concerned with Olympic-style athletic feats. Remember that if you are out of shape, your peers may be as well. While many Americans no longer make time for community sports, you can be among the exceptions. You can make playing shortstop on that community softball team a pursuit that lasts many years. Longevity and variety are the name of the game.

You can achieve variety through shorter bursts of exercise as well. Frequent, short bouts of exercise increase fat burning. You can split up your exercise sessions into two daily 20-minute aerobic sessions as opposed to a single 40-minute cycling or swimming session. The separate power sessions will fit into your schedule and give you renewed octane levels to fuel your day. Recent research from Canada's research-intensive McMaster University, published online in the *American Journal of Physiology*, indicates that short bursts of high-intensity sprints improve the structure and function of blood vessels as much as traditional longer-duration exercises.

If you think this all sounds good but you worry that you can't stick to a plan, use positive mental imagery. Take time to visualize yourself engaging in regular exercise and developing a fitter body that is ready to fight disease and to help you pursue your dreams.

Yes, Exercise Does Benefit You

The majority of people know that keeping physically active and exercising regularly are both good for your health. This is why so many people resolve on New Year's Eve to "exercise more." However, when you become as specific as you can about your exercise plan, you'll see a difference. Following the fitness recommendations in Chapter 2 has been proven to do the following:

1. Lower blood pressure
2. Decrease the risk of heart disease related to high blood pressure
3. Fight off type 2 diabetes
4. Aid in weight control
5. Improve circulation
6. Increase bone strength
7. Reduce the risk of certain types of cancer

Since item number one on the list is the focus of this book, let's talk specifically about how exercise lowers blood pressure. As we saw in the study on Wesley in Chapter 2, experts don't know specifically what magic exercise works. One obvious answer is that exercise helps weight loss, which eases the strain on blood vessels. And if you participate in cardiovascular aerobic exercise, it is likely you will see reductions in "resting" blood pressure, or the level of systolic and diastolic pressure while you rest, which is important for most of us! Cardiovascular aerobic exercise includes the entire body, and the goal is to raise the heart rate and sustain it throughout the workout time. Thirty minutes of cardiovascular aerobic exercise will result in increased heart volume and oxygen consumption, improved blood circulation, and enhanced metabolism.

However, you don't have to work particularly hard or exercise all day to see results in lowering your blood pressure. Doctors accept that all forms of exercise seem to lower blood pressure, although most studies agree aerobic exercise is slightly more effective for people who have high blood pressure. My experience validates these conclusions.

How does regular exercise reduce blood pressure? There seem to be a few different ways. Perhaps most importantly, exercise affects the sympathetic nervous system and decreases resistance to blood flow in the blood vessels. In addition, exercise increases the kidneys' elimination of sodium, which subsequently reduces fluid volume and then ultimately blood pressure.

Research evidence indicates that regular exercise training, which means exercise activity three or four times per week, decreases resting systolic blood pressure in individuals with high blood pressure. After at least one month, people who exercise three or four times a week will likely see a drop in resting systolic blood pressure. Also, while shorter periods of 30 minutes do a world of good in lowering blood pressure, if you increase your amount of low- to moderate-intensity physical activity from 30 to 45 minutes on most days of the week, you may even see a greater reduction in blood pressure. Specifically, regular aerobic exercise done for extended periods is an important component of a medical treatment plan for most people with mild high blood pressure. Of course, this is something to discuss with your doctor! We also now know that with extended periods of regular moderate-intensity exercise, significant changes are seen not only in blood pressure but also in cholesterol and other risk factors for heart disease.

We've mentioned low-, moderate-, and vigorous-intensity exercise. Although moderate exercise is generally recommended, lower levels of *intensity* may certainly be helpful in lowering blood pressure. *Circulation*, a journal of the American Heart Association, has reported that nine months of low-intensity exercise has produced a systolic decrease of 20 mmHg and diastolic decrease of 12 mmHg respectively in older high-blood-pressure patients. These results are remarkable! Other studies have also shown promising results.

And the research continues to unfold! Hormone studies link high insulin levels and insulin resistance, in which insulin is impaired, with high blood pressure. Other studies state that aerobic exercise—which once again has a slight edge over other forms of physical activity—can reduce insulin levels and insulin resistance in people with high blood pressure. Also, exercise reduces adrenaline, also known as the fight-or-flight response hormone, while endorphins give you that "exercise high" that makes you feel better overall. Your heart rate slows down and your circulation doesn't work as hard.

Exercise and Aging

As I've mentioned, blood pressure tends to increase with age. Regular exercise inhibits or even reverses this trend and many of the other declines commonly associated with aging. A long-term regimen of three to five brisk 30-minute walks or other 30-minute physical activities each week, for instance, may not only add years to your life, but experts believe it may also add vitality to your years.

Major universities are now conducting similar studies into the effects of exercise on high blood pressure in American children (the other end of the spectrum). The benefits of exercise for young people have been amply documented, as has the absolute need for increased physical activity for our children. The most I can say within the scope of this book is that, as with adults, the amount of exercise, rather than the intensity, is more important in keeping a healthy blood pressure in children. It is not a coincidence that childhood rates of obesity and high blood pressure have increased in recent years and are higher than ever before. This phenomenon has somewhat paralleled the decrease in exercise and physical activity over the past 50 years as outside activity is often stolen away by video games and computers. For younger and older people alike, exercise lowers blood pressure. However, special populations such as very obese people can especially benefit. The key takeaway here is that exercise *does* reduce blood pressure for most people, no matter which group you may fall into.

What's Your Fitness Level?

Let's talk about *how* to exercise properly to reduce high blood pressure. Most of our discussion will center on aerobic and cardiovascular exercise, which, as we've mentioned, generally involves at least 20 minutes of exercise.

We'll break down the topic further and address your specific exercise needs at your level of proficiency. I have not made any assumptions as to your fitness level. According to my experience, the readers of this book fall into one of four categories:

a. Expert/Advanced—they are already fit, but maybe need some coaching
b. Work-Fit—they do a great deal of physical activity for work/as a parent but not at any other time
c. Barely Fit—they are sedentary because of jobs, commutes, and hobbies; have difficulty keeping a routine; rarely exercise on their own and have physical difficulty doing so; are over 50 and have gotten out of the habit; may have heart problems
d. Beginner—they want to exercise but are convinced it's complicated

Most healthy people don't need to see a doctor before the start of moderate exercise, but I do recommend you check with your physician or a guaranteed fitness expert for guidance. On the other hand, those with high blood pressure should always follow a doctor's recommendations. Remember, you are not looking for a short-term quick fix for your blood pressure . . . that doesn't exist. As your mother might say, "Get out and play, but don't end up in the emergency room." Take it slow at first.

Here are some specific precautions to take when embarking on an exercise program. For example, if you like to run, be careful with running on asphalt—try to find padded tracks if running outdoors; also, swimming, bicycling, and elliptical training are excellent modes of exercise to deter joint arthritis. Be careful with power lifting and sudden, jerking-type movements to avoid injury. Of course, power lifting has its place in athletic competition, but gives a low "return on investment" for most outside of elite athletes and may in fact lead to more injuries.

At one time, I weighed approximately 185 to 190 pounds and I routinely "threw up" (as they say) approximately twice my body weight on the free-weight bench press and three times my body weight on the squat rack when training for football. I gave this up, however, when I tore my rotator cuff for the second time in my late twenties. I reasoned that I had a lot of time to enjoy the benefits of exercise, and I didn't want to lose out on exercise because of injury and pain. How many pro athletes have you seen who trained for sports but ended their careers because of injuries that could have been avoided? If it happened to them, it can definitely happen to you, particularly if you're out of practice. It's certainly fine and motivational to set fitness goals, but stay within reasonable limits for the best results.

To avoid injury, I suggest some universal guidelines. Every workout should begin with five to seven minutes of warm-ups followed by light stretching and breathing exercises. Begin slowly and gradually work up to a light perspiration. This is important if you follow the recommendation for 30 minutes of completely aerobic cardiovascular exercise. Even cross-training exercises or circuit-training equipment such as the elliptical trainer can have great cardiovascular benefit. However, warming up before you begin circuit training will help your heart rate and ease you into the rhythm and speed of your workout.

Go, Speed, Go

This brings me to another question I regularly get: How do you know what speed to use during the aerobic portion of your workout?

Well, we have already made some mention of intensity. Aerobic exercise is not a drag race, but rather the Indy 500 or the Daytona 500. If you pace yourself properly, you won't run out of gas. You can pace yourself by measuring your heart rate often during your workout. You'll also gauge the intensity of your efforts. Remember, the difference between moderate- and vigorous-intensity activities is the increased heart rate. This will help you avoid overworking your heart—you want the heart muscle to be exercised, not exhausted. There is a simple equation to estimate your maximum heart rate.

Don't be scared of the word "equation." This is not trigonometry. Just take your age and subtract it from the number 220. For example, Wesley in Chapter 2 is 55, so 220 − 55 equals 165. This is Wesley's maximum heart rate, as shown in Table 5.4. Then, you figure out 50 to 85 percent of this number, and the result is known as your target zone. Wesley calculated his range as 83 to 140. This range is where everyone should normally be during the exercise.

Table 5.4. Average Maximum Heart Rate by Age

Age	Target Heart Rate Zone 50–85% (beats/minute)	Average Maximum Heart Rate 100% (beats/minute)
20 years	100–170	200
25 years	98–166	195
30 years	95–162	190
35 years	93–157	185
40 years	90–153	180
45 years	88–149	175
50 years	85–145	170
55 years	83–140	165
60 years	80–136	160
65 years	78–132	155
70 years	75–128	150

When you start an exercise program, you will do well to follow the American Heart Association suggestion that you aim at the lowest part of your target zone, 50 percent, during the first few weeks. You can gradually build up to the upper range of your target zone, such as 75 percent. After six months or more of regular exercise, you may be able to exercise comfortably at up to 85 percent of your maximum heart rate. The study Wesley participated in backed up this assertion. However, maintaining at least 70 percent is plenty adequate to stay in shape. Certain conditions and blood pressure medications may prevent you from safely increasing your heart rate, so again, please discuss this with your medical doctor.

If these calculations are still a bit cumbersome, Table 5.4 shows average estimated target heart rates for different ages. Look for the age category closest to yours, and then read across to find your target heart rate.

What if you can't measure your pulse or just don't want to take your pulse when exercising? The American Heart Association says to try the "talk and walk" method. If you can talk and walk at the same time, you aren't exerting yourself too hard. If you can sing or hum along to your favorite music and maintain your level of effort, you aren't working hard enough. If you get out of breath quickly, if you have to stop and catch your breath, you need to roll back on the intensity. Always, always breathe if you are working out for prolonged periods and during high-intensity sessions of 20 minutes. Holding your breath during aerobic exercise can raise blood pressure to dangerous levels.

Shorter and Faster

I think this leads into a good opportunity to discuss anaerobic exercise, so I will spend a few moments on the topic. Anaerobic just means exercise that is short lasting, but of high intensity and power output. I have to caution readers that this type of exercise is not particularly beneficial for blood pressure and/or cardiovascular health.

When many think of being fit, they think of large, densely muscled bodybuilder types, such as California's "Mr. Universe" and Governator Arnold Schwarzenegger. However, the man once known as "The Austrian Oak" also served as former President George H. W. Bush's chairman of the President's Council on Physical Fitness. One of his main political initiatives as governor was to launch the Council on

Physical Fitness and Sports, a nonprofit organization established to promote making California the nation's "Fitness State." His speeches and writings on exercise after his bodybuilding career emphasize aerobic activity as well as weight training. He has come to understand what doctors have confirmed. Anaerobic bodybuilding that builds lots of muscle mass isn't directly related to good health at all, since less body mass generally equates to better health. Also, blood pressure may become extremely elevated during intense resistance training. Blood pressure measurements during resistance suggest readings can become dangerously high.

I don't mean that you should forget strengthening exercises, but as you may have already guessed, strength training works best as part of a comprehensive program.

All of this assumes that you are mobile and not hindered by arthritis or obesity. If you do face physical limitations, don't assume you can skip exercise altogether.

Help for the Exercise-Challenged

In a perfect world, no one would have any difficulty with exercise. However, we know that this is not the case in reality. For example, although walking is the most universally effective means of exercise, there may be many of you out there who experience difficulty with walking, especially due to conditions affecting the major walking joints such as the knees and the hips. Fortunately, there are very few conditions in which walking may actually be detrimental (such as when acute bone fractures are present, etc.). Many people in their fifties and sixties who don't have acute bone fractures may not be able to jog but can enjoy a brisk stroll. If you experience any discomfort when walking, it is very important to talk to your doctor about it so that a sound solution and/or alternative may be implemented. You may be able to substitute swimming, a non-weight-bearing activity that benefits arthritis sufferers. Swimming is wonderful for people with arthritis because the body is supported by water. Joint pressure is lessened in the water, allowing more freedom and flexibility of movement. Doing water aerobics or swimming energizes the body and makes you feel good. It's an excellent way to exercise even if you can't engage in weight-bearing activities.

When you hear the words "weight bearing," some of you may have the image of muscle-bound bodybuilders (for example, Schwarzenegger) lifting barbells. More simply, this means that exercise is done on your feet, which support your weight as you exercise. Bone adapts to the impact of weight and the pull of muscle by building more bone cells. Consequently, bone becomes stronger and denser, which reduces bone loss from osteoporosis and decreases the risk of fracture. Common weight-bearing activities include:

- walking
- jogging
- hiking
- dancing
- step aerobics
- basketball
- tennis
- golf
- stair climbing

Many arthritis patients with moderate-to-severe physical limitations will look at the list of weight-bearing exercises and regrettably be able to participate in few or none of the activities. Patients with mild symptoms should be able to do more.

Walking or playing golf for people with high blood pressure and mild arthritis may be a challenge, but the irony is that avoiding weight-bearing exercise, or for that matter, any exercise, may actually do *more* harm. A sedentary lifestyle means you are sitting or resting most of the time. A sedentary lifestyle is not healthy. For people with arthritis, sedentary is definitely not the way to go. Being sedentary increases blood pressure and works to increase perceived pain in weight-bearing joints such as the knees and hips. Remember the feeling you have when you get up after hours sitting at a desk studying or working? That stiffness can become painful for the person whose only exercise involves walking to the car for the drive home, then walking to the television to collapse. Before long, that person experiences pain at the slightest movement. Arthritis may take root, and even more pain follows. Obesity, depression, and difficulty sleeping feed on this pain and increase it further. Because pain may cause a person to become less active, and less activity increases pain, a terrible cycle can ensue.

Exercise breaks that cycle! Studies have shown that exercise helps people with arthritis in many ways. Exercise reduces joint pain, inflammation, and stiffness and increases:

- flexibility
- muscle strength
- cardiac fitness
- endurance
- weight control

Weight control may be especially important for people with arthritis, because obesity and abdominal fat can place strain on joints and increase inflammation. Therefore, I recommend an exercise plan that takes your limitations into account but still is effective.

It may be difficult for people with arthritis to stick with a regular exercise program because of their physical limitations. Therefore, it's important for arthritis sufferers to learn about the different types of exercise before deciding on fitness goals and plans and discussing those plans with a doctor and physical therapist or athletic trainer. Your doctor will know which types of exercise are not appropriate and may make a referral to a physical therapist or athletic trainer. It is best to find a physical therapist that specializes in or has experience working with people with arthritis. Your physical therapist ideally will be familiar with pain-relief methods, proper body mechanics (placement of the body for a given task), joint protection, and energy conservation.

I have consulted with physical therapists. Based on their recommendations and my own conclusions, I can confidently state that if you have arthritis, the following types of exercises are appropriate to incorporate into your routine with proper supervision:

1. Range-of-Motion Exercise

Physical therapists follow a doctor's prescription and lead patients through gentle stretching exercises that move each joint—for example, knee, hip, and shoulder—as far as possible in all directions. These exercises are crucial for people with joint conditions, particularly since normal, everyday routine activities do not take joints through the full range of motion. Gentle stretching routines can be done daily and should be done at least every other day to help maintain normal joint movement, relieve stiffness, and increase flexibility.

2. Strengthening Exercise

You use light hand weights and possibly ankle weights to work your muscles. You can progress from three-pound weights to five-pound weights and eventually ten-pound weights and beyond. Working your triceps, biceps, pectorals, and deltoids will improve strength and muscle tone throughout your body. You can also perform squats, lifts, and lunges while you hold hand weights, but follow the guidance of your therapist. Strong muscles help support and protect joints affected by arthritis. If you have severe pain or swelling in your joints, avoid this type of exercise. If your joints are reasonably healthy and you have mild pain or discomfort, you can perform strengthening exercises every other day to improve joint function. If your joints become swollen, painful, or red, consult your doctor immediately.

3. Aerobic Exercise

We've already covered aerobic exercise extensively in this chapter, but arthritis sufferers may think that aerobic activity is beyond their abilities. Unless you have severe pain or swelling in your joints, you can and should perform the aerobic activities already mentioned in this chapter for 20 to 30 minutes three times a week. Remember that 20- to 30-minute exercise routines can be performed in increments of 10 minutes over the course of a day.

These are general guidelines. Your physical therapist, athletic trainer, and doctor can further explain the exercises to you. Be sure to ask what types of exercise are safe for you to do, how often you should be doing the exercises, and why it's important to consistently participate in some form of exercise on a regular basis. People with arthritis should discuss exercise options with their doctors and other health care providers. Many people with arthritis begin with easy, range-of-motion exercises and low-impact aerobics.

You may also want to ask what the right amount of activity is for your situation. Not everyone is exactly the same, so you have to evaluate your activity level on an individual basis. Physical activity or exercise should always begin gradually to determine what level is best for you, so that you can find a balance between too much activity and too little. If you find that your body pain is heightened the day after a range-of-motion or strengthening exercise session, you probably did too much exercise at a level above your physical tolerance.

The amount and form of exercise recommended for each individual with arthritis will vary, depending on such factors as which joints are involved, the level of joint inflammation, how stable the joints are, and/or whether a joint replacement procedure has been done. In order to sustain the strengthening associated with weight-bearing exercise, the intensity, duration, and amount of stress applied to bone should increase over time. But arthritis patients with physical limitations may have a problem with increasing the intensity of exercise. In addition, high blood pressure can reinforce the limitations placed upon you by joint pain.

If you are dealing with joint pain and blood pressure, I recommend a plan for lowering your blood pressure that you can implement as you embark on your exercise program. My plan for lowering blood pressure in people with joint problems includes:

- Medical supervision
- Rest and relaxation
- Proper diet
- Medication
- Instruction on other pain relief methods
- Instruction on ways to conserve and maintain your energy
- Information on the protection of joint muscles
- Instruction on proper body mechanics (placement of the body during exercise)

Research into exercise will continue to be important for people with high blood pressure as well as joint conditions. My colleagues and I often search for and find benefits from exercise for patients with high blood pressure and joint conditions.

As you lower your blood pressure and strengthen your joints, you can expand your exercise program, assuming your doctor approves. People with arthritis can participate in a variety of, but not all, sports and exercise programs with the benefit of a support system of people working toward similar fitness goals. Many community centers, health clubs, and hospitals offer fitness programs and classes tailored to people who have arthritis or other physical limitations. Working with a group can combat the problem of motivation that deters many people with arthritis from exercising.

You will still need to expend effort and energy and invest time in exercise. Your investment may be greater and more gradual than if you did not have arthritis. However, the return on investment will make your dedication worthwhile.

Let's recap the general plan for exercising with arthritis:

1. Discuss exercise plans with your doctor.
2. Get supervision from a physical therapist or qualified athletic trainer.
3. If you need to increase joint comfort, apply heat to sore joints (many people with arthritis start their exercise program this way).
4. Stretch and warm up with range-of-motion exercises.
5. Start strengthening exercises slowly with small hand and/or ankle weights (three to five pounds).
6. Progress slowly.
7. If you need to ease joint pressure, use cold packs after exercising (many people with arthritis complete their exercise routine this way).
8. Add aerobic exercise.
9. Ease off if joints become painful, inflamed, or red. Work with your doctor to find the cause and eliminate it.
10. Choose the exercise program you enjoy most and make it a habit. Join community exercise classes to help you stay on track.

As mentioned, you can consider appropriate recreational exercise after you start with structured range-of-motion, strengthening, and fitness-center aerobic exercise. Fewer injuries to joints affected by arthritis occur during recreational exercise if it is preceded by range-of-motion, strengthening, and aerobic exercise that gets your body in the best condition possible.

Some of you may think that these goals seem too demanding, especially if you are still employed, juggling family responsibilities, and battling physical hardships. As people continue to work past the age of retirement, for financial and personal reasons, older workers will increasingly struggle with arthritis and high blood pressure. Younger workers, including those with families, also strive to be healthy despite limited personal time and exponentially increasing physical difficulties. Younger people seem to be more and more susceptible to high blood pressure than was thought in the past. They are also not immune from arthritis or joint problems. In an ideal world, people would get flextime to take care of fitness, and some companies do address this need. However, in an increasingly competitive and unpredictable economy, you can't take an arthritis day or exercise day off from work, so the exercise dilemma of people who work deserves attention.

When Exercise Isn't Part of the Job Description

Many of us work in jobs that exercise our minds (or not!) but keep our bodies sedentary, such as data processing, laboratory analysis, information technology, toll booths, and so on. Even business travelers often don't have flexibility to exercise, since they are on someone else's schedule, sitting in meetings, and riding on planes. And often, employers may not budget for a hotel with a 24-hour fitness center.

The irony is, however, that having out-of-shape employees with arthritis, obesity, and high blood pressure costs employers dearly in lost productivity. Employers depend on sedentary workers, especially in today's technology-driven workplace, and business travel. It's worth diverting from our emphasis on patients with arthritis and mobility issues to answer another question I frequently get asked: "How can I exercise during my workday or when I am traveling?"

Staying Fit for Stationary Workers

Many people work in jobs in which they sit all day, then rush home to prepare dinner, keep a house, and attend to children and spouses. By the time office workers come home from a long commute and handle all the daily responsibilities, there is little energy left for exercise. Stealing time for exercise during the day may seem unrealistic, but it may be the optimal time for most office and sedentary workers to do it.

Building and maintaining strength and tone in our abdominal muscles and core, which refers to our upper torso, is a big concern for computer-based workers and secretaries, who often sit in uncomfortable positions for hours on end. Even doctors such as radiologists spend hours reading images on a computer screen at workstations. I have heard of doctors in other hospitals setting up treadmills under workstations. This is expensive, especially when doctors have to rotate shifts. Most companies don't allow for such investments, but I would certainly encourage these healthy environmental modifications.

If you are sedentary at work, you can still squeeze in some exercise. For example, taking the stairs to your office may help your fitness level. I have received many suggestions from people who use creativity to exercise when there's no treadmill, fitness class, or gym.

- Keep a pair of weights underneath your desk or in a drawer.
- If you have your own office and you can work privately for an hour or so, sit on an exercise ball. As you move back and forth on the ball, it gently helps work your abs, core, glutes, and thighs.
- Do mini abdominal crunches while you're sitting in your chair. Contract the abdominal muscles and then release them. Do this rapidly several times in a row.
- Do seated calf raises, which will strengthen your joints and calf muscles, with less pressure on feet and ankles than standing calf raises. **Seated calf raises are especially beneficial if you have an ankle injury.**
- Do seated stretches to increase your flexibility.
- Get up and move about for three to five minutes every hour you sit. Walk to someone's office instead of phoning, e-mailing, or text messaging.

Every business setting is slightly different, so it is important to incorporate fitness that works with the company culture and job obligations.

Advice for Business Travelers

Anyone who travels for business, even within a city on sales calls, knows that although you're out of the office, your opportunities to exercise may still be limited. Most sales calls or site visits aren't conducive to fitness. Perhaps you can keep a set of hand weights in the trunk of the car and do strengthening exercises to clear your mind before making a presentation. It does take creativity. Salespeople aren't on a regular schedule, and they are at the mercy of their employers and clients. Don't let this compromise your health.

Similarly, the majority of long-distance business travelers must conform to someone else's budget and time. When business travelers aren't in airports, in cars, or at meetings, they may have free time, but the hotel may not have a gym with a 24-hour open schedule. Many hotel gyms are sparsely equipped with few hand weights, without weight machines, and with one or two aerobic machines that always seem to be busy. The hotels that do have pools usually keep them open for limited hours.

Many business travelers are able to exercise during breaks or "downtime" at a conference or a day filled with meetings. Here are some suggestions to create your own exercise-on-the-go plan.

- Because of airport security, it may not be wise to pack hand weights in carry-ons. However, if you have a long layover or airplane delay and you use the business lounge, you can even do moderate aerobic routines if the lounge isn't crowded.
- Pack small weights or a jump rope in your checked baggage.
- Take the stairs at the hotel. Climbing flights of stairs will clear your head and help you sleep better so you feel more rested when you have to get up for that 6 a.m. presentation.
- If your meetings start later in the morning or end early in the evening, consider making use of the hotel pool.
- Don't pass up golfing outings and other business-sponsored athletic activities. They are ideal networking opportunities, and you can keep your body in good condition while you pursue business opportunities.

Talk to your doctor and fitness trainer—they may have some knowledge and insight into staying fit on the road when you can't follow a structured exercise program. Few health professionals, however, will doubt that you are well advised to follow some type of exercise program, even if it's unconventional.

Workers with more latitude who can incorporate regular gym activity and need a detailed program can benefit from the sample regimen I've devised for an on-the-go or less-busy lifestyle.

Comprehensive Sample Program

Now we come to the most-asked question after "What is the best exercise book?" Groups always ask me what the best workout is for people who are reasonably healthy but who have high blood pressure and weight-control issues. Although there is not just "one workout that fits all," some general and complete workout routines can be considered. It is important to discuss with your doctor whether or not a program is appropriate for you.

Here is a sample program that you may consider with your health professional. You may want to gradually add these exercises, and some may not be appropriate for everyone. If you are not familiar with the weight machines listed in the workout, ask a gym instructor or staff member how to use each machine.

My program focuses on incorporating adequate aerobic exercise with muscle-strengthening exercises. Of course, the amount of weight used and the intensity of the workout vary from person to person. If time becomes a constraint, be sure to make the aerobic portion (e.g., Precor machine) a priority.

Day 1

These exercises focus on chest and triceps muscles (push exercises). It's important that you use the therapeutic bands to strengthen rotator cuff muscles.

Exercise	Reps or Minutes
Pre-Cycle 1	
Precor EFX (machine)	7 min.
Chest Stretch	3 min.
Abdominal Crunch (machine)	15
Arm Inward Rotation (bands)	12
Arm Outward Pull (bands)	12
Cycle 1	
Seated Chest Press (machine)	12
Triceps Extension (machine)	12
Seated Pec Fly (machine)	12
Reverse Straight-Arm Flys (machine)	12
Abdominal Crunch (machine)	15
Cycle 2	
Arm Inward Rotation (bands)	12
Arm Outward Pull (bands)	12
Seated Chest Press (machine)	12
Triceps Extension (machine)	12
Seated Pec Fly (machine)	12
Reverse Straight-Arm Flys (machine)	12
Abdominal Crunch (machine)	15
Precor EFX (machine; moderate)	30 min.

Day 2

Today's exercises focus on back and biceps (pulling exercises), and place a little more emphasis on abdominal muscles.

Exercise	Reps or Minutes
Pre-Cycle 1	
Precor EFX (machine)	7 min.
Biceps Stretch	3 min.
Spinal Twist Stretch	2 min.
Squatting Lat Stretch	3 min.
Cycle 1	
Abdominal Crunch (machine)	15
Seated Lat Pulldown (machine)	12
Seated Lat Row (machine)	12
Biceps Curl (machine)	12
Back Extension (machine	12
Torso Rotation (machine)	12
Abdominal Crunch (machine)	15
Leg Raise	15
Cycle 2	
Seated Lat Pulldown (machine)	12
Seated Lat Row (machine)	12
Biceps Curl (machine)	12
Incline Chest Raise (machine)	12
Torso Rotation (machine)	12
Abdominal Crunch (machine)	15
Incline Leg Pull-In (machine)	12
Precor EFX (machine; moderate)	30 min.

Day 3

Find time to do at least 30 minutes of physical activity such as mowing the lawn, walking, tennis, biking, golfing (without a cart), and so on—whatever you would like.

Day 4

Focus on chest and triceps as in Day 1 but with less weight and more repetitions (e.g., 15 instead of 12).

This day incorporates some specific exercises for leg muscles, although each day your legs are certainly getting some exercise through the aerobic cycles.

Again, using the bands to strengthen rotator cuff muscles is very important—the cuff consists of four tiny muscles that can easily be damaged if not properly stretched and strengthened.

Exercise	Reps or Minutes
Pre-Cycle 1	
Precor EFX (machine)	7 min.
Chest Stretch	3 min.
Hip Flexion Stretch	4 min.
Arm Inward Rotation (bands)	15
Arm Outward Pull (bands)	15
Abdominal Crunch (machine)	15
Cycle 1	
Seated Chest Press (machine)	15
Triceps Extension (machine)	15
Seated Pec Fly (machine)	15
Seated Leg Press (machine)	15
Abdominal Crunch (machine)	15
Hip Abductor (machine)	15
Hip Adductor (machine)	15
Lying Leg Curl (machine)	15
Seated Calf Raise (machine)	15
Arm Inward Rotation (bands)	15
Arm Outward Pull (bands)	15
Cycle 2	
Seated Chest Press (machine)	15
Tricep Extension (machine)	15
Seated Pec Fly (machine)	15
Seated Leg Press (machine)	15
Hip Abductor (machine)	15
Hip Adductor (machine)	15
Lying Leg Curl (machine)	15
Seated Calf Raise (machine)	15
Abdominal Crunch (machine)	15

Day 5

This is similar to Day 2, but with higher repetitions.

Exercise	Reps or Minutes
Pre-Cycle 1	
Precor EFX (machine)	7 min.
Biceps Stretch	3 min.
Spinal Twist Stretch	2 min.
Squatting Lat Stretch	3 min.
Abdominal Crunch (machine)	15
Cycle 1	
Seated Lat Pulldown (machine)	15
Seated Lat Row (machine)	15
Biceps Curl (machine)	15
Back Extension (machine	15
Torso Rotation (machine)	15
Abdominal Crunch (machine)	15
Leg Raise	15
Cycle 2	
Seated Lat Pulldown (machine)	15
Seated Lat Row (machine)	15
Biceps Curl (machine)	15
Incline Chest Raise (machine)	15
Abdominal Crunch (machine)	15
Incline Leg Pull-In (machine)	15
Precor EFX machine (moderate)	30 min.

Day 6

You can perform 60 to 90 minutes of physical activity such as mowing the lawn, walking, tennis, biking, golfing (without a cart), and so on.

Day 7

Rest and/or enjoy light physical activity as in Day 3 and Day 6.

This program is comprehensive yet geared to complement the schedules and lives for people who have family and career obligations as well—in other words, most adults. My rule of thumb is to plan to exercise at least four days out of every week so that it becomes a habit. One suggestion is to plan to go to the gym.

The primarily goal during the actual workout is to keep things moving. Don't let anything break the flow of exercise. Resting on a machine, or pausing too long while exercising, compromises the workout benefit by reducing intensity and lengthening the time the workout takes.

Notice that in this sample workout, there are no back-to-back sets of the same exercise. This practice is known as circuit training, in which you move between exercise machines amid sets. Although circuit training has been around for some time, it has lost attention in fitness settings. Have you ever waited as someone paused between sets on a machine? It's counterproductive, and can even seem rude, unless you are elderly or disabled. As a rule, most relatively healthy adults need only a brief rest between sets in a cycle, about the time it takes to walk to the next exercise. However, after you complete a cycle, rest a little bit longer, for one to two minutes, before starting the next cycle. The goal is to complete the entire workout generally in about an hour or less. Some people will need a few minutes less, while others, at a different fitness level, will need more time.

I would recommend gradually working into the full program, especially if you are not accustomed to exercise or if you need to use caution because of your blood pressure levels. Be sure to take your blood pressure readings before, after, and during the workout. Pausing to check your blood pressure is not rude or counterproductive; it's sensible.

What if you want to work your abdominals? Low-impact lower abdominal exercises can help add tone to your core. You can always add on abdominal exercises at the end of the routine if they are not already included. However, you will notice that there is at least some work on the abdominals every day. Abdominals are core muscles and very important for stability. They can be worked most days of the week, including through walking.

However, while you improve your physical condition, you can increase physical activity levels in your life, even when you're not at the gym. Every little bit helps. Ask the tortoise in the classic fable. The tortoise beat the hare through slow, gradual progress. You may not think you're doing anything exercise related at a given time, but every moment offers opportunities to move, flex, and strengthen. As you saw in Table 5.2 and Table 5.3, common chores can help you in the pursuit of fitness.

What About "Doing Dishes": A Fitness Trend?

I mentioned that exercise is more satisfying than doing the dishes. However, you can incorporate physical activity into everyday moments. Weed, trim, and rake the lawn and garden and you may burn up to hundreds of calories. An old-fashioned hand lawn mower may burn even more calories! Table 5.5 has figures on calories spent in activities. You'll notice that the more a person weighs, the more calories are burned.

Find out how many calories are burned during common tasks, and if you can't do your favorite activity—for example, swimming—you don't have to miss out on the benefits of movement. At the same time, you can help your blood pressure and your garden grow through spading dirt, lifting bags of soil, and tilling the soil. Don't look at these tasks as chores but opportunities to get even healthier! This attitude should help you work more energetically at a constant pace.

Worldwide, chores could be the new fitness craze in the future, but not yet! The *American College of Sports Medicine (ACSM) Health and Fitness Journal* has come out with the Top Worldwide Fitness Trends for 2009 as shown in Table 5.6.

Outcome measurements are of particular interest here when we consider exercise for blood pressure reduction. For example, instructors of mindful exercise such as yoga have suggested that people enrolled in t'ai chi, qigong (pronounced "chi-gong"), and yoga classes have blood pressure readings taken at four- to six-week intervals during the classes. Mindful exercise emphasizes awareness of your breath, your body, and your muscles. The goal of mindfulness is for you to be able to turn off your anxious thoughts, including ones about your blood pressure readings, and be in the present moment whatever you are doing. This is good for your entire body and has the effect of reducing stress. As we'll see in Chapter 8, reducing stress prolongs your life and brings down blood pressure, which is the outcome you desire, whether you are doing weight lifting or mind/body exercise.

It may seem odd to talk about measuring outcomes and mind/body exercise in the same paragraph, but they can work together. You are aware of your exercise goals, but not anxious over them, which will make your exercise routine seem less daunting. This is of tremendous benefit when your main goal is to exercise to lose weight to feel better, look better, and lower your blood pressure.

Many of you at this point probably want to learn how to exercise to lose weight. After all, maintaining a healthy weight is a cornerstone of

Table 5.5. Calories Burned in 1 Hour of Activity

Activity	100 lbs.	120 lbs.	140 lbs.	160 lbs.	180 lbs.	200 lbs.	220 lbs.	240 lbs.	260 lbs.	280 lbs.	300 lbs.
Aerobic dancing (low impact)	115	138	161	184	207	230	253	276	299	322	345
Aerobics, moderate effort	145	174	203	232	261	290	319	348	377	406	435
Aerobics, slide training (basic)	150	180	210	240	270	300	330	360	390	420	450
Basketball (game)	220	264	308	352	396	440	484	528	572	616	660
Basketball (leisurely, non-game)	130	156	182	208	234	260	286	312	338	364	390
Bicycling, 10 mph (6 minutes/mile)	125	150	175	200	225	250	275	300	325	350	375
Bicycling, 13 mph (4.6 minutes/mile)	200	240	280	320	360	400	440	480	520	560	600
Golfing (walking, w/o cart)	100	120	140	160	180	200	220	240	260	280	300
Golfing (with a cart)	70	84	98	112	126	140	154	168	182	196	210
Hiking with a 10-lb. load	180	216	252	288	324	360	396	432	468	504	540
Hiking with a 20-lb. load	200	240	280	320	360	400	440	480	520	560	600
Hiking with a 30-lb. load	235	282	329	376	423	470	517	564	611	658	705
Hiking, no load	155	186	217	248	279	310	341	372	403	434	465
Jogging, 5 mph (12 minutes/mile)	185	222	259	296	333	370	407	444	481	518	555
Jogging, 6 mph (10 minutes/mile)	230	276	322	368	414	460	506	552	598	644	690
Racquetball	205	246	287	328	369	410	451	492	533	574	615
Rowing (easy)	75	90	105	120	135	150	165	180	195	210	225

(continued)

Table 5.5. *(continued)*

Activity	100 lbs.	120 lbs.	140 lbs.	160 lbs.	180 lbs.	200 lbs.	220 lbs.	240 lbs.	260 lbs.	280 lbs.	300 lbs.
Rowing machine	180	216	252	288	324	360	396	432	468	504	540
Running, 8 mph (7.5 minutes/mile)	305	366	427	488	549	610	671	732	793	854	915
Running, 9 mph (6.7 minutes/mile)	330	396	462	528	594	660	726	792	858	924	990
Running, 10 mph (6 minutes/mile)	350	420	490	560	630	700	770	840	910	980	1050
Soccer	195	234	273	312	351	390	429	468	507	546	585
Stair–climber machine	160	192	224	256	288	320	352	384	416	448	480
Stair climbing	140	168	196	224	252	280	308	336	364	392	420
Swimming (25 yards/minute)	120	144	168	192	216	240	264	288	312	336	360
Swimming (50 yards/minute)	225	270	315	360	405	450	495	540	585	630	675
Tennis	160	192	224	256	288	320	352	384	416	448	480
Tennis (doubles)	110	132	154	176	198	220	242	264	286	308	330
Volleyball (game)	120	144	168	192	216	240	264	288	312	336	360
Volleyball (leisurely)	70	84	98	112	126	140	154	168	182	196	210
Walking, 2 mph (30 minutes/mile)	60	72	84	96	108	120	132	144	156	168	180
Walking, 3 mph (20 minutes/mile)	80	96	112	128	144	160	176	192	208	224	240
Walking, 4 mph (15 minutes/mile)	100	120	140	160	180	200	220	240	260	280	300
Weight training (40 sec. between sets)	255	306	357	408	459	510	561	612	663	714	765
Weight training (60 sec. between sets)	190	228	266	304	342	380	418	456	494	532	570
Weight training (90 sec. between sets)	125	150	175	200	225	250	275	300	325	350	375

Table 5.6.   ACSM 2009 Top Worldwide Fitness Trends

1. Educated and experienced fitness professionals
2. Children and obesity
3. Personal training
4. Strength training
5. Core training
6. Special fitness programs for older adults
7. Pilates
8. Stability ball
9. Sport-specific training
10. Balance training
11. Functional fitness
12. Comprehensive health promotion programs at the worksite
13. Wellness coaching
14. Worker incentive programs
15. Outcome measurements
16. Spinning (indoor cycling)
17. Physician referrals to fitness professionals
18. Exercise and fitness programs
19. Group personal training
20. Reaching new markets

Source: Walter R. Thompson, Ph.D., FACSM, FAACVPR, *ACSM Fitness and Health Journal*, Vol. 12, No. 6.

staying fit. Some of the advice about weight loss and exercise currently available may confuse you as you aim for your goals, so it's worthwhile to take a little time to explore some of the myths you may have heard about or grown up with.

Exercise, Weight Loss, and Blood Pressure

Let's return to Table 5.5 for a moment. I have been asked, "Dr. Rhoden, maybe I should weigh more so that I will burn more calories during activities and therefore lose more weight." Well, of course this is a little silly, since being heavier means that you have a lot more calories to lose, and it takes many calories to equal a pound. The idea is to reduce your weight and your blood pressure sensibly. Take in less than you burn, and burn more than you take in.

On that note, try to avoid programs that encourage weight loss without exercise. The combination of diet and exercise interventions has been shown significantly more effective than diet or exercise alone in the treatment of obesity. If you just restrict eating without changing your physical habits, it is difficult to win control of your weight. Many people wonder why the blood pressure readings don't improve much during a new diet. You could eat the blandest foods without salt or caffeine, you could try a miracle shake at lunch and dinner, but if you don't exercise, you may only minimally improve your health or your blood pressure, and you most likely won't lose weight. However, I will share a secret: Exercising in conjunction with weight loss works best to improve blood pressure.

As we've seen, regular exercise has heart health benefits, and those can't be measured solely by changes in weight. We spoke in Chapter 2 about motivation and putting your emphasis on staying active. You'll find your exercise far more enjoyable and effective if you focus on the positive benefits that occur throughout your body: less insulin resistance, decreased stress, decreased blood pressure, and slower aging to a point. Focus on these, not on what your scale says or those extra pounds that keep you from your target weight. A sound weight-control and exercise program does not use scale weight as the only marker of success. If your doctor or personal trainer doesn't understand the health benefits of exercise beyond weight loss, you may want to consult someone that does.

In my presentations to groups, I have heard the grim tale of a health care provider who, in the course of giving treatment for high blood pressure and heart disease, approached the person's weight in a less-than-sensitive or helpful manner. Some patients who sought help for weight loss may have felt blamed and not helped by doctors. In my mind, the subject of weight should always be brought up respectfully. It is an important factor in health and can be changed. However, excess weight is such a hot button that it evokes powerful reactions, however unfairly, from the people who possess the excess weight and the individuals around them. This adds stress for people who are trying to lose weight. Society's expectations, to say nothing of our own, can push our efforts in an unhealthy direction.

Our drive diminishes before the pounds do, whether we are on a proven weight-loss program or a fad diet. Even on the best weight-loss programs, you can get discouraged when you assume that your efforts have yielded little benefit. Keep in mind that the healthiest weight-loss goals are for the long term and generally defined as one year or longer. Remember that in the fable "The Tortoise and the Hare," the tortoise didn't need any fancy tricks or shortcuts to reach the finish line. Unfortunately, in our lives we're surrounded by people who are fast, lean, and flashy, like the hare. They're in the media, on magazines, on television, in our social groups, and in the workplace. When you get discouraged by these images, think of your motivation for exercising and losing weight, and don't compare yourself with other people.

On the surface, your weight is certainly different from your blood pressure. After all, you can't see blood pressure by looking at someone. A number of studies have found that several harmful "inflammatory" factors decline when people exercise and lose weight. Being overweight contributes to fat tissue that is metabolically active and produces hormones and chemicals that harm the cardiovascular and other systems. Fat tissue that accumulates in the midsection and expands our waistlines is especially active or volatile like fire. This tissue can become "ignited," also known as inflammation, and the effect is similar to pouring gasoline on fire. You can think of the fires in the body, the inflammation, being put out by weight loss.

It's meaningful that exercise, even without weight loss, has been shown to reduce both waist size (an easy-to-measure approximation for dangerous abdominal fat) and one of the chemicals produced by fat tissue. A sensible weight management program will eliminate fat tissue and conserve lean tissue that burns calories instead of storing them. A sensible program will help direct you to lose weight necessary to reduce the risk of heart disease and high blood pressure.

The amount of weight loss needed to improve your health may be much less than you wish to lose when you consider how you personally evaluate your weight. If I suggest an initial weight goal that seems too small for you, please understand that my major emphasis is on your health. I also want you to know that your health can be greatly improved by a loss of only 5 to 10 percent of your starting weight. It doesn't guarantee that you will reach your ultimate goal weight, as this may differ from person to person, but you will be making a monumental improvement in your health. You'll decrease your body mass index and reduce other obesity-related problems. A reduction of 5 to 10 percent doesn't mean you have to stop there. An initial goal of losing 5 to 10 percent of your starting weight is both realistic and valuable.

What does such a program look like for people who sit behind a desk all day, or whose daily workout consists of walking to the mailbox? As I mentioned, weight loss and management all comes down to energy balance: calories in (from food and drinks) versus calories out (from daily activity and exercise). If weight loss is your goal, you need to eat fewer calories than you use on a daily basis. For example, a calorie decrease of 500 per day will lead to a loss of one pound per week. Even a calorie deficit of 100 calories per day will help, since Americans gain about two pounds per year. Eating an extra 100 unnecessary calories can lead to a weight gain of ten pounds per year on average—and this is not uncommon!

Let's say you want to burn 100 calories and/or eliminate 100 calories from your diet every day. There are many ways to do this, and here are some suggestions. Think of these as my 100-calorie-pack suggestions.

Part A: Burn 100 calories when you . . .

- Walk for 30 minutes
- Shovel snow for 15 minutes
- Climb stairs for 15 minutes
- Do general housework for 25 minutes

As we've seen, you can avoid monotony and feel as if you are accomplishing something special with ordinary chores if you mix it up. Alternate sports and exercise with physical activities we do all day without thinking about them.

Part B: Cut at least 100 calories from your diet if you . . .

- Eliminate one tablespoon of butter or margarine
- Replace eight ounces of regular soda with diet soda or another noncaloric drink, such as water
- Have an apple instead of a single-serving bag of chips
- Switch from a bakery bagel to a two-ounce small, frozen bagel
- Have half a cup of ice cream instead of a cup

Burning or eliminating 100 calories may not sound like a lofty goal or a particularly meaningful one. After all, we have the mind-set in this culture that everything should be big, dramatic, and immediately measurable. We are success oriented. However, burning 100 calories through exercise adds up over time, contrary to what many exercise program promoters would have you believe. All you need is a firm commitment every day to cut 100 calories or to burn 100 calories. Focus on that goal with regularity for a week, then a month, then a year, until it becomes second nature.

Some exercise programs promise results with perhaps only a month of time investment. However, consistency is the key to fitness. You can make it like clockwork—just as you have a set period for lunch or a set meeting of the parents' association, the sales team, or both, you can schedule an exercise appointment, even in the middle of the workday. Besides your lunch break, you have other opportunities where you work. Workplace fitness and gyms have cropped up thanks to the overall losses of productivity and revenues that are directly related to employees' high blood pressure and obesity. Many workplaces even have fitness classes and allow employees to exercise while "on the clock."

It may be helpful to keep a fitness diary in which you record the time and duration of exercise. One entry might be, "Played basketball on employee basketball court for 30 minutes." It may be helpful to record your blood pressure before and after the workouts, to chart the relationship between your exercise habits and your blood pressure readings. You will get a sense of accomplishment from charting your progress. Experts highly recommend the exercise diary in addition to other motivational tools. You can chart where you let your exercise habits fall by the wayside, which will happen. You can learn, through an exercise journal, to be patient with yourself and focus on your successes rather than your failures. You can also reward yourself along the way—although not with a big steak and mashed potatoes, which will just negate the positive effect of the exercise! For example, you may write, "My BP measurement was down to 128/65 after this week of exercise. Reward: a trip to the movies or a concert."

You can use the fitness diary to record your visualizations of your desired outcomes. Focus on your successes, not your missteps! Reaffirm your weight loss goals, or that goal to burn 100 extra calories every day. You will see results! My goal with all of the above information is to give you a road map through a maze of misinformation, distractions, and obstacles. My goal is also to inspire you. You can become more fit despite all the challenges. Just consider this story . . .

Donna's Story

Donna had not exercised since her freshman year of college, and her weight had ballooned to 270 pounds. She occasionally took an aerobics class but ended up so sore and out of breath that she felt discouraged. She tried Pilates but could never find even 10 minutes for herself to do a workout.

Donna is a successful information technology consultant who crams ten hours of work into an eight-hour day at a firm that constantly demands top performance. Then, Donna goes home to her husband and daughter after she takes care of any errands that need to be run. Donna's days barely leave her time to breathe or even eat properly. In the past, when she or her husband picked up their seven-year-old daughter and then came home from work, the family's mealtime ritual involved takeout or microwaveable and prepackaged foods.

For several years Donna struggled with her weight, and she increasingly noticed that her daughter showed signs of childhood obesity. Donna knew the situation was far from healthy, but she felt stuck in that pattern. Then one day she felt dizzy when she got up from her chair at her workstation. The next thing she knew, she was lying on the floor and one of her colleagues had called 911.

Donna learned she had high blood pressure. She didn't want to believe the elevated BP reading taken by the doctor she consulted. She got a second opinion from a doctor at our hospital that confirmed the first reading. In addition, Donna had insulin resistance, and she confessed to the second doctor that she was experiencing joint pain. She feared she was developing arthritis at age 37. Her doctor prescribed exercise, high blood pressure medication, and a complete diet overhaul. Donna was concerned that she wouldn't be able to follow an exercise regimen. She sought advice from her doctor, who recommended several chair exercises that office workers can do during the course of a normal workday. It was also recommended that Donna and her family pick a healthy activity to do together. Donna's daughter and husband liked to roller skate, so the whole family decided to try Rollerblading.

Donna struggled with the changes but grew to enjoy the seated ab exercises, which became popular in her department as information technology workers attempted to improve their fitness. Donna's abdominal fat began to disappear. She also did weight-bearing exercises and supplemented walking with trips to the pool with her daughter. Donna delegated some of her work responsibilities and was able to leave work earlier one day a week so that she and her daughter could swim together at a community pool.

Donna was able to drop 120 pounds in ten months. She now feels much better at 150 pounds, which is still not her ideal weight. Her doctor developed a diet plan that included a set schedule and easy-to-prepare meals she could plan every week. Donna accepts the daily intake of 1,000 calories, and surprisingly her family has adjusted without feeling deprived. Her husband has reported that he too was becoming overweight, but now feels much better. Donna's daughter has nipped her childhood obesity in the bud and frequently reminds her mother to exercise and eat fresh vegetables. She is proud that her mother exercises most days of the week for at least 30 minutes.

Donna hopes to increase her workout time to an hour even if she has to grab 10-minute intervals throughout the day. Her exercise has eased her joint pain, and she may avoid the onset of arthritis. Her blood pressure has dropped below the high normal range. In addition, she is aiming for a healthy maximum weight loss of one to two pounds per week now that her dramatic weight loss has tapered off. Donna is pleased that she has been able to customize her weight loss and exercise plan. This has made all the difference in her ability to follow a diet and exercise regimen.

Following the Plan

Sticking to your exercise goals can sometimes be difficult. Sometimes we "fall off of the wagon," so to speak. As we've seen, it's easy to get discouraged when the numbers don't tell us what we want. You can discipline you mind to focus on what's important. Dropping 10 pounds immediately is not as important as feeling more fit and having more energy.

Going forward, you may reach a point where you find it somewhat difficult to adhere to the exercise program you've laid out for yourself. This scenario does not always signify weakness or faintheartedness. It simply means we're only human. On occasion, you may encounter troublesome circumstances where such factors as time constraints and conflicting priorities may cause you to second-guess your decision to exercise. Keep in mind that the difficulties and obstacles of today are the cost of the accomplishments of tomorrow. You are making a change that goes against years of habits. So hang in there. Your body is undergoing changes that may not always be readily apparent until you take that blood pressure reading or walk up the stairs without feeling out of breath.

You may feel guilty taking time out for yourself, but your loved ones will probably understand the message of that cartoon I spoke of in the beginning. Your loved ones certainly don't want you to collapse and die one day without warning. Make exercise a priority, for your sake and theirs. Remember the safety card on airplanes? The instructions tell you that if the aircraft cabin is depressurized and oxygen masks drop down, you need to inflate and secure your own mask before you help others. You need to be physically and mentally well to meet all the challenges of your life and to help the people who count on you.

Equally important, you deserve to feel good! In order to sustain an active lifestyle, it is certainly important to find activities you enjoy. If joining the gym sounds like torment, you're probably not going to go with any enthusiasm. Having enthusiasm will turbocharge your workout. That way, when you plan specific attainable goals, such as "I will play tennis for 30 minutes three times a week, and if I can't do that I'll dance to my favorite music, alone or in a group," you'll look forward to dancing or tennis. If you include other people in your scheduled activities, you have a support system of people who enjoy the same activity. Make sure that your goals are reasonable in terms of financial and time investment. If you can't afford to play tennis or go dancing, then schedule an alternate activity: "I will walk for 20 to 30 minutes before work on Monday, Wednesday, and Friday."

If you can't do the whole workout, remember that doing something is better than doing nothing. If you can't get in your regular 45-minute workout, use the 20 minutes you do have. You will be surprised how much better you feel after only 20 minutes of aerobic activity. This is the additive effect. If you do 20 minutes of aerobic activity four times a week or more at a reasonable level, you will be in very good muscular and cardiovascular shape. Your blood vessels will thank you. Your heart will thank you.

Exercise is a potent antidote to high blood pressure. As I've said, lifestyle changes such as improved diet and increased physical activity will also work in conjunction with high blood pressure medications to bring down those blood pressure numbers. As the medications work, your lifestyle changes will help save your life by bringing down your blood pressure to the ideal number!

Now that we've tackled the topic of exercise and blood pressure, let's turn to the burning questions you have about high blood pressure medication. Although the following chapter will by no means be all-inclusive and the only source you should use as reference, I certainly hope that it will help!

Chapter 6

THE ROLE OF MEDICATION IN BRINGING DOWN HIGH BLOOD PRESSURE

WE HAVE TALKED ABOUT the importance of taking steps to keep your blood pressure under control. The treatment goal is blood pressure below 120/80 and can potentially be even lower for certain conditions such as diabetes and kidney disease. Essentially healthy people report that adopting healthy lifestyle habits is sufficient to control high blood pressure in most cases.

Treating high blood pressure without medication is certainly desirable. However, when lifestyle changes alone are not effective in keeping your pressure controlled, it may be necessary to add blood pressure medications. In some cases, diet and exercise may not be enough.

Adoption of a healthy lifestyle is critical in managing and treating high blood pressure. As we have already mentioned, exercise is a wonderful way to reduce blood pressure. Weight reduction as well as diet modifications, such as the ones I have given or the DASH Diet, are also an indispensable part of managing high blood pressure. For example, according to the Seventh Report of the Joint National Committee on Prevention, Detection, Evaluation, and Treatment of High Blood Pressure (JNC 7), a DASH eating plan that limits sodium intake to 1,600 mg a day is as effective as taking a single high blood pressure drug. Combining two or more lifestyle modifications such as the JNC 7 recommendations listed in Table 6.1 can work even better.

The JNC 7 report provides several key recommendations for the overall treatment and management of high blood pressure. These recommendations include benchmarks to measure the severity of high

Table 6.1. JNC 7 Lifestyle Recommendations to Reduce High Blood Pressure

Modification	Recommendation	Approximate SBP* Reduction Range
Weight reduction	Maintain normal body weight (BMI = 18.5–25)**	5–20 mmHg/10 kg weight lost
DASH eating plan	Diet rich in fruits, vegetables, low-fat dairy, and reduced-fat	8–14 mmHg
Restrict sodium intake	<2.4 grams of sodium per day	2–8 mmHg
Physical activity	Regular aerobic exercise for at least 30 minutes most days of the week	4–10 mmHg
Moderate alcohol	≤2 drinks/day for men and ≤1 drink/day for women	2–4 mmHg

*SBP = systolic blood pressure
**BMI = body mass index

Source: Chobanian, A. V. et al. *Journal of the American Medical Association* 2003; 289: 2560–72.

blood pressure, which in turn are used to determine the need for medication. The JNC 7 benchmarks state that:

- In people older than 50, systolic blood pressure greater than 140 mmHg is a more important cardiovascular disease (CVD) risk factor than diastolic blood pressure.
- People with high normal blood pressure at age 55 have a 90 percent lifetime risk for developing high blood pressure.
- The risk of CVD beginning at 115/75 mmHg doubles with each increment of 20/10 mmHg.
- Individuals with a systolic blood pressure of 120 to 139 mmHg or a diastolic blood pressure of 80 to 89 mmHg should be considered pre–high blood pressure; they require health-promoting lifestyle modifications to prevent CVD.

The recommendations most relevant to this chapter are:

- Many individuals, especially those with diabetes or chronic kidney disease, will require two or more high blood pressure drugs for control.
- Thiazide-type diuretics are usually recommended for patients who have high blood pressure without complications.
- There are compelling reasons to prescribe other classes of drugs (angiotensin-converting enzyme inhibitors, angiotensin receptor blockers, beta-blockers, calcium channel blockers) for high blood pressure patients with certain high-risk conditions.
- If blood pressure is significantly high (over 20/10 mmHg above target high blood pressure), doctors consider beginning drug therapy with two agents, one of which is typically a thiazide-type diuretic.

A question I hear frequently is, "When do you know if you absolutely need medication?" This depends on your blood pressure rating. I base my recommendations on how high your blood pressure readings are and what your high blood pressure risk factors are, your associated cardiovascular risk factors, whether or not you have heart disease (most critical), and whether or not you have damage to other organs.

I usually follow the classification of heart disease from the evaluation system in the sixth Joint National Committee's report on the Prevention, Detection, Evaluation, and Treatment of High Blood Pressure (JNC 6). The rating system is known as the JNC 6 Risk Stratification System, which is provided in Table 6.2.

People in risk group A:

- Have normal blood pressure in the upper normal limit, *or* stage 1, 2, or 3 high blood pressure without other risk factors and without organ damage or clinical cardiovascular disease.
- Can first undergo lifestyle modification with frequent blood pressure monitoring in stage 1 high blood pressure. If the target blood pressure isn't achieved within one year, doctors should add drug treatment.
- Are treated with medication in stage 3 high blood pressure.

Table 6.2.   JNC 6 Risk Stratification System by Risk Group

Your Blood Pressure	Risk Group A	Risk Group B	Risk Group C
130–139/85–89 High normal	Lifestyle modification	Lifestyle modification	Drug therapy
140–159/90–99 (called stage 1 high blood pressure)	Lifestyle modification (up to 12 months)	Lifestyle modification (up to 6 months)	Drug therapy (up to 6 months)
≥160/≥100 (Called stages 2 & 3 high blood pressure)	Drug therapy	Drug therapy	Drug therapy

Adapted from Table 5 from *The Sixth Report of the Joint National Committee on Prevention, Detection, Evaluation, and Treatment of High Blood Pressure (JNC 6)* NIH Publication #98-4080, November 1997; National Heart, Lung and Blood Institute, National Institutes of Health.

Most people with high blood pressure fall into risk group B. People in risk group B:

- May have a number of risk factors other than diabetes.
- Do not show any evidence of organ damage or clinical cardiovascular disease.
- May need drug treatment initially, depending on the blood pressure stage and number of high blood pressure risk factors.
- Will need lifestyle modification, as with all the risk groups.

People in risk group C are most in need of prompt drug therapy as well as lifestyle modifications. They include:

- Patients with high or high normal blood pressure.
- People who have clinical evidence of target organ damage, clinical cardiovascular disease, and/or diabetes, with or without risk factors.

The JNC 7 and I agree that the most effective drug regimen prescribed by the most conscientious and careful doctor only controls high blood pressure if you as the patient are motivated. I know from experience that doctor empathy for a patient and positive doctor-patient experiences are powerful motivators. Make sure you trust your doctor. This is increasingly important if you are at greater risk and need medication.

I Need Medication—What Do I Do Now?

Treating high blood pressure requires patience and care from both doctor and patient. It may be annoying to take pills and possibly have side effects, especially if you felt fine before treatment. Don't be discouraged if you must be treated with medication and take more than one blood pressure–lowering medication. Often two or more drugs are more effective than one.

Some people can reduce their drug dosages after achieving normal blood pressure and maintaining it for a year or more. Be advised, however, that you shouldn't make any changes without first discussing them with your doctor. Taking blood pressure medication may be frustrating; however, coping with the inconvenience of medication is still much better than suffering a stroke or heart attack.

If you have to take high blood pressure medication, especially if you are taking it for the first time, you are probably looking for in-depth information about blood pressure medications.

The ABCs of Blood Pressure Drugs

Another question groups ask me most frequently is, "Which medication is best?" There is certainly no simple answer to this question. I will endorse no particular medication brand in this book.

It would take a large pharmacologic textbook to detail every bit about blood pressure medications, and to weigh the merits exhaustively. However, this chapter will give a general rundown of the main types of blood pressure–lowering drugs. These are the drugs most commonly prescribed and recommended. I'll also reveal how these medications work.

If you know the "ABCDEs," you will be well on your way. I'll list all the classes of drugs and provide the generic drug names. The generic drug names for a particular class of drug all have the same ending, such as –pril and –artan.

Angiotensin-Converting Enzyme (ACE) Inhibitors

Brand Name (Generic Name): Lotensin (benazepril), Capoten (captopril), Vasotec (enalapril), Monopril (fosinopril), Prinivil, Zestril (lisinopril), Univasc (moexipril), Aceon (perindopril), Accupril (quinapril), Altace (ramipril), Mavik (trandolapril)

What They Do: ACE inhibitors are used to lower blood pressure in people with heart failure and people with high blood pressure. These drugs prevent the formation of a hormone called angiotensin II, which normally causes blood vessels to narrow. The drugs cause the vessels to relax and expand the vessels to decrease resistance. As blood pressure goes down, the heart works more easily and efficiently.

ACE inhibitors are a very effective "class" of medication for many people. That said, health care providers often prefer these medications for people with diabetes. This is because the medication has fewer side effects, does not affect blood sugar levels, and provides additional kidney protection.

Cautions: Be aware that your health care provider may perform blood tests to make sure there are no effects on your potassium levels or kidneys in conjunction with this medication. Ask your health care provider about these tests.

Your doctor should not prescribe ACE inhibitors if you are pregnant or are planning to become pregnant. If you do take ACE inhibitors and discover you are pregnant, talk to your doctor about switching to another drug.

Side Effects: Be sure to always report anything you think may be a side effect to your physician. All medications come with information inserts. It is important to familiarize yourself with this detailed information. However, it is also important to remember that some individuals may react differently to medications than others. Be aware of possible side effects. Bear in mind that just because the effect is on the label, that certainly doesn't mean it will happen to you.

Side effects of ACE inhibitors include dry cough, rash, or itching; allergy-like symptoms; allergic reaction with generalized swelling; and excess potassium in the body, especially in people with kidney failure.

Angiotensin-II Receptor Antagonists (ARBs)

Brand Name (Generic Name): Atacand (candesartan), Teveten (eprosartan), Avapro (irbesartan), Cozaar (losartan), Micardis (telmisartan), Diovan (valsartan)

What They Do: ARBs have been shown to produce effects similar to those produced by ACE inhibitors. ARBs shield blood vessels from angiotensin II. As a result, the vessels become wider and blood pressure goes down. In addition, rather than lowering levels of angiotensin II (as ACE inhibitors do), angiotensin II receptor blockers prevent this chemical from having any effects on the heart and blood vessels. This keeps blood pressure from rising.

Like ACE inhibitors, this type of blood pressure medication is commonly prescribed for people with diabetes, because of the extra protection provided for the kidneys.

Cautions: There is controversy over whether ARBs such as Valsartan increase the risk of myocardial infarction. There is not yet any confirming evidence to support this claim, but controversy remains thanks to some study results.

Your doctor should not prescribe ARBs if you are pregnant or are planning to become pregnant. If you do take ARBs and discover you are pregnant, talk to your doctor about switching to another drug.

Side Effects: ARBs do produce cough less frequently than ACE inhibitors and may be tolerated better. However, some of the most common side effects of this type of medication include dizziness/lightheadedness, decreased kidney function, and increased potassium levels.

Beta-Blockers

Brand Name (Generic Name): Tenormin (atenolol), Kerlone (betaxolol), Ziac (bisoprolol/hydrochlorothiazide), Zebeta (bisoprolol), Cartrol (carteolol), Sectral (acebutolol), Lopressor, Toprol XL (metoprolol), Corgard (nadolol), Inderal (propranolol), Betapace (sotalol), Blocadren (timolol)

What They Do: Beta-blockers essentially produce low blood pressure because they reduce nerve impulses to the heart and blood vessels. This makes the heart beat more slowly and with less force. Blood pressure drops and the heart works more efficiently.

Cautions: It is important not to stop taking this type of medication abruptly without a medical doctor's supervision.

Beta-blockers may increase the effects of medications such as other high blood pressure drugs, insulin, muscle relaxants, and some antidepressants.

Beta-blockers may cause increased breathing difficulty in people who have asthma or hay fever. For people with diabetes, beta-blockers may hide some of the warning signs of low blood sugar. If you have diabetes and you take a beta-blocker, your heart rate may not increase in response to a low blood sugar level. You will need to check your blood sugar levels carefully after you start taking a beta-blocker.

You may ask why there have been a few references to diabetes in this chapter. Well, we talked in an earlier chapter about the fact that it may be of even greater importance to control blood pressure in people with diabetes. Also, blood pressure problems are also commonly found in persons with diabetes.

Side Effects: Insomnia, cold hands and feet, fatigue, depression, slow heartbeat, symptoms of asthma.

A Note on Beta-Blockers and Exercise: I have been asked whether people should be careful when exercising and taking beta-blockers or whether exercise eliminates the need for this medication. Beta-blockers reproduce the natural effects of exercise. They lower your heart rate and blood pressure. However, exercise doesn't give you some of the side effects of beta-blockers, which reduce aerobic fitness by 10 percent.

This is not to say that you should automatically go off your medication just because you have started doing aerobic exercises. Exercise typically works together with medication. A study published in the June 2007 *American Journal of Physiology: Heart and Circulatory Physiology* found that exercise training together with beta-blockers improved heart health and circulation in older adults.

Calcium Channel Blockers (CCBs) or Calcium Antagonists

Brand Name (Generic Name): Norvasc, Lotrel (Amlodipine), Vascor (bepridil), Cardizem, Tiazac (diltiazem), Plendil (felodipine), Adalat, Procardia (nifedipine), Nimotop (nimodipine), Sular (nisoldipine), Calan, Isoptin, Verelan (verapamil)

Note that in the case of CCBs, the generic names do not always have the same endings, as there are actually different classes within this overall category. You'll notice that the majority of generic names in the category end in –ipine.

What They Do: CCBs "interrupt" the movement of calcium into heart and blood vessel muscle cells. This relaxes the blood vessels, and blood pressure drops. Besides being used to treat high blood pressure, they're also used to treat angina (chest pain) and/or some arrhythmias (abnormal heart rhythms).

There are short-acting and long-acting CCBs. Short-acting CCBs work relatively fast, but their effects last only a few hours. Long-acting CCBs start working gradually, but their effects last longer.

Cautions: Amlopidine has a minimal effect on heart rate and contraction. It is safer than other CCBs for people with high blood pressure who also have a slow heart rate or heart failure. On the other hand, verapamil powerfully slows down the heart and is recommended for people who have an abnormally fast heart rate. The National Heart, Lung and Blood Institute has advised doctors that "short-acting nifedipine should be used with great caution (if at all), especially at higher doses, in the treatment of high blood pressure, angina, and myocardial infarction."

CCBs are typically not recommended for people with heart failure, low blood pressure, heart rhythm problems, heart or blood vessel conditions, or other structural damage to the heart. People who have Parkinson's disease, a history of depression, kidney or liver disease, low blood sugar, or food allergies should be careful when taking CCBs.

CCBs are more often prescribed for younger people than for people over 60, and reservation is used for pregnant women as well as women who are breastfeeding.

Many medicines interact with food. Good examples are verapamil and nifedipine, which interact with grapefruit. This interaction reduces the liver's ability to eliminate the drugs from the body. Therefore, these medications shouldn't be taken with grapefruit or grapefruit juice because the grapefruit juice can cause the medications to build up in your body. Wait at least four hours after you have taken your medication before you drink grapefruit juice. Alcohol also interferes with the effects of CCBs. Don't smoke while you take CCBs, since tobacco can cause a rapid heartbeat (among other things!)

Tell your doctor if you are taking any of these medications that can intensify or decrease the effects of CCBs:

- Other high blood pressure medications, in particular beta-blockers and ACE inhibitors, diuretics, and digitalis.
- Medicines to treat an irregular heartbeat.
- Corticosteroids or any cortisone-like medicines.
- Certain eye medications.
- Large doses of calcium or vitamin D supplements.

Side Effects: Constipation, headache, rapid heartbeat, rash, drowsiness, nausea, swelling in the feet and legs, fever, chest pain, shortness of breath, fainting, wheezing and coughing, flushed face and skin, dizziness, constipation, and heartburn. Many of these side effects are seen as side effects of other medications as well.

Diuretics/"Water Pills"

Brand Name (Generic Name): Midamor (amiloride), Bumex (bumetanide), Diuril (chlorothiazide), Hygroton, Thalitone (chlorthalidone), Lasix (furosemide), Esidrix, Hydrodiuril (hydrochlorothiazide), Lozol (indapamide), Aldactone (spironolactone), Dyrenium (triamterene)

As you can see, most diuretics end in –ide or –one. There are many different types of diuretics, distinguished from each other by their methods of action. Diuretics are among the oldest drugs used to treat high blood pressure.

What They Do: Diuretics are sometimes called "water pills" because they work in the kidney and "flush" excess water and sodium from the body tissues, lowering blood pressure. Many of you probably have a family member that talks about that "water pill" causing frequent trips to the bathroom. Or in fact, maybe you have experienced this effect yourself. It is certainly true. The more excess water and sodium diuretics flush from your system, the more often you have to go to the bathroom. Some of these medications, however, may have a greater effect on urination than others.

According to information from the National Institutes of Health, generic thiazide diuretics such as chlorthalidone, hydrochlorothiazide, and indapamide may be just as important as more expensive blood-pressure-lowering drugs in reducing blood pressure. Furthermore, thiazide diuretics have been shown to prevent heart attack, heart failure, and stroke in people with metabolic syndrome, a condition that affects millions of Americans and makes them more susceptible to type 2 diabetes. In the past, people with diabetes have been advised to use caution when taking diuretics because of increased blood sugar levels. However, it is now consistently recommended that thiazide diuretics should be the first choice for most people with high blood pressure, especially patients with metabolic syndrome or type 2 diabetes. Patients that can't take this drug may need other types such as ACE inhibitors, ARBs, and CCBs. Also, sometimes diuretics alone don't bring the desired effects, so they may be combined with other blood pressure medications.

Cautions: Ask your doctor about the effects the medicine you are taking has on nutrients. For example, most diuretics cause your body to get rid of calcium, but a certain type actually causes your body to "hold on" to calcium.

Some diuretics may decrease your body's supply of potassium, which of course we mentioned earlier in the nutrition and blood pressure chapter. Eating foods containing potassium may help prevent significant potassium loss caused by these drugs. You can prevent potassium loss by taking a potassium liquid or tablet together with your diuretic, if your doctor recommends it. However, certain diuretics such as spironolactone can actually increase potassium levels.

To reduce side effects and make the drug more effective, limit salt and increase intake of potassium-rich produce in addition to low-fat dairy and whole grains. For the first three to six months you take the drug, rise slowly from lying to standing. Avoid prolonged sun exposure and drink lots of water during exercise. Exercise frequently. If you have stomach flu or any illness causing diarrhea or vomiting, stop taking diuretics and call your doctor. Also see your doctor if you experience severe muscle weakness as well as numbness or tingling in the fingers and around the mouth.

Take your blood pressure readings at home and insist that your doctor test your calcium, cholesterol, glucose, sodium, and potassium levels at regular intervals. For example, before you start the drug, one month after you begin medication, then once or twice a year.

Ask your doctor about pain relievers while you are also taking diuretics because of an increase in the diuretic effects with drug-to-drug interaction. Also, lithium can quickly become toxic when you take diuretics. People with diabetes who take insulin and diuretics at the same time should be wary of increases in the potency of both insulin and diuretics.

Side Effects: Fatigue, leg cramping, and increase in blood sugar, LDL cholesterol, and triglycerides. A high level of triglycerides in the blood is often a sign of other conditions that increase your risk of heart disease (such as metabolic syndrome).

Extra Medication Types/Nitroglycerin

We have already discussed briefly the most commonly used medications for high blood pressure. If you are aware of these medications, then you are certainly a very savvy health care consumer, especially with regard to pharmaceuticals for blood pressure. On the other hand, some medications are less commonly prescribed but may be used in certain situations, most often when the common medications are not tolerated well and/or additional medication is needed to control blood pressure.

1. Alpha Blockers

Brand Names (Generic Names): Uroxatral (alfuzosin), Cardura (doxazosin), Dibenzyline (phenoxybenzamine), Regitine (phentolamine), Minipress (prazosin), Flomaxtra/Flomax (tamsulosin), Hytrin (terazosin)

What They Do: This class of drug reduces nerve impulses to blood vessels, which allows blood to pass more easily, causing the blood pressure to go down.

Cautions: Alpha blockers are not typically used as the drug of choice but may be in certain situations (e.g., benign enlargement of the prostate).

Alpha blockers are generally taken at bedtime. Additionally, the risk of a "first dose phenomenon" may be reduced by starting at a low dose and titrating upward, or increasing dosage, as needed. Because these medications may cause low blood pressure, the agents may interact with other medications that increase risk for low blood pressure.

Side Effects: Low blood pressure that may lead to dizziness, light-headedness, or fainting when rising from a lying or sitting posture.

2. Nitroglycerin/Nitrate Vasodilators

Brand Names: Nitro-Bid, Nitro-Dur, Nitrostat, Transderm-Nitro, Minitran, Deponit, Nitrol any creative forms of nitroglycerin medication have been developed, including extended-release capsules, ointment with tape for application, patches, translingual spray (through the tongue), and sublingual tablets (under the tongue), as well as cheek (buccal) tablets.

What They Do: Nitrates act to correct the imbalance between the flow of blood and oxygen to the heart and the work the heart must do by dilating the arteries and veins in the body. Nitroglycerin medications relax the smooth muscle in blood vessels, causing them to dilate, which reduces the amount of blood that returns to the heart to be pumped. Dilation of arterial blood vessels brings about a drop in blood pressure in the arteries against which the heart must pump, so that the heart works less hard and requires less blood and oxygen.

Think of nitroglycerin as a heart relaxer or soother. This medication is typically used for chest pain caused by angina pectoris, or chest pain as a result of heart disease, but has been proven effective in lowering blood pressure.

Cautions: All medications should be stored at proper temperatures; however, storage for this particular type of medication requires some special attention. All formulations should be kept at room temperature, 59 to 86°F (15 to 30°C). The sublingual tablets are especially susceptible to moisture. Nitroglycerin medications should not be kept in bathrooms or kitchens because of the higher degrees of moisture there, and care should be taken to replace the sublingual tablets every six months.

It is very important to remember that interactions with other drugs are especially dangerous with nitroglycerin. Like alpha blockers, nitroglycerin can cause low blood pressure. Other medication you may be taking that also causes hypotension, for example other high blood pressure medications, antidepressants, antipsychotics, and antianxiety drugs, may produce an unwanted additive effect. Anti-migraine medicines and over-the-counter decongestant pseudoephedrine medications (e.g., Sudafed) may interfere with the actions of nitroglycerin.

Since alcohol also may intensify the blood-pressure-lowering effect of nitroglycerin, patients taking nitroglycerin are advised to drink alcoholic beverages with extreme care.

To reduce the risk of low blood pressure, patients often are told to sit or lie down during and immediately after taking nitroglycerin.

Side Effects: A persistent, throbbing headache, flushed skin, and increased heart rate.

NOTE: We won't list every type of blood pressure medication, although keep in mind there are some additional types, including those used in emergency situations. An exhaustive compendium is not important. It is vital, however, to know that sometimes your physician will prescribe more than one anti-high-blood-pressure medication. These medications often work synergistically and are known as combination therapies.

Combination Therapies

The anti-high-blood-pressure medications on the market are similar in their overall effectiveness in lowering blood pressure, although individual responses may vary. Different strategies help to select the best single drug for a patient. However, surveys of hospitals around the nation indicate that many patients are taking more than one anti-high-blood-pressure medication.

In practice, few high blood pressure patients can reach their target blood pressure with monotherapy, which means a single drug therapy. Epidemiologic studies, however, have shown that a high percentage of individuals on medication using only a single drug do not reach the target level of less than 140/90 mmHg. By today's standards, even this level is inadequate for most high blood pressure patients with several additional risk factors, such as chronic kidney failure. In general, most people with high blood pressure require treatment with two or more anti-high-blood-pressure agents to achieve optimal blood pressure control. It has been suggested that since the cutoff point between "normal" and "high" blood pressure is being pushed increasingly downward, especially for patients with multiple cardiovascular risk factors, most high blood pressure patients need more than one drug to reach their target blood pressure.

Drug combinations have multiple advantages. The cost may actually be lower. Consumers and doctors alike often find combination therapies convenient, since there are, surprisingly, fewer pills to take. Combination therapies allow lower doses of individual drugs. Although the downsides of combination drug therapies may include a loss of flexibility (patients are "locked" into specific doses and drugs) as well as increased potential for adverse reactions that may not always have a clear cause, patients find combinations of drugs easier to tolerate, and patients are more inclined to take combinations of drugs, so compliance with a doctor's direction is increased. Patients accept lifelong drug therapy more easily with combination formulations of drugs.

Common combinations of various types of anti-high-blood-pressure drugs include:

- ACE inhibitors and calcium channel blockers (CCBs)
- ACE inhibitors and diuretics
- Angiotensin receptor blockers (ARBs) and diuretics
- Beta-blockers and diuretics
- CCBs and beta-blockers
- Hydrochlorothiazide (HCTZ) and thiazide diuretics ("water pills")

Table 6.3 details common fixed-dose combinations of specific drugs.

Table 6.3. Commonly Prescribed Drug Combination Therapies

Hydrochlorothiazide (HCTZ) drug combinations

- Clonidine + HCTZ (*Clorpres*)
- Hydralazine + HCTZ (*Hydra-Zide*)

Diuretics

- HCTZ + spironolactone (*Aldactazide, Al-tazide, Al-daciazinc*)
- HCTZ + amiloride (*Moduretic*)
- HCTZ + triamterene (*Dyazide, Maxzide*)

ACE inhibitor + diuretic

- Benazepril + HCTZ (*Lotensin-HCT*)
- Captopril + HCTZ (*Capozide*)
- Enalapril + HCTZ (*Vaseretic*)
- Lisinopril + HCTZ (*Zestoretic, Prinzide*)
- Quinapril + HCTZ (*Accuretic*)
- Moexipril + HCTZ (*Uniretic*)
- Fosinopril + HCTZ
- Perindopril + HCTZ
- Fosinopril + HCTZ
- Perindopril + HCTZ
- Ramipril + HCTZ

ARB + diuretic

- Losartan + HCTZ (*Hyzaar*)
- Irbesartan + HCTZ (*Avalide*)
- Valsartan + HCTZ (*Diovan-HCT, Co-Diovan*)
- Eprosartan + HCTZ (*Teveten-HCT*)
- Telmisartan + HCTZ (*Micardis-HCT*)
- Candesartan + HCTZ (*Atacand-HCT*)
- Olmesartan + HCTZ (*Benicar-HCT*)

Beta-blocker + diuretic

- Atenolol + HCTZ (*Tenoretic*)
- Propranolol +HCTZ
- Nadolol + bendroflumethiazide (*Corzide*)
- Bisoprolol +HCTZ (*Ziac*)
- Timolol + HCTZ (*Timolide*)

(continued)

Table 6.3. (*continued*)

ACE inhibitor + CCB

- Benazepril + amlodipine (*Lotrel*)
- Trandolapril + verapamil SR (*Tarka*)

CCB + beta-blocker

- Nifedipine + atenolol

Source: I. Gavras, and T. Rosenthal "Combination Therapy as First-Line Treatment for Hypertension." *Current Hypertension Reports* 2004, Aug., 6(4): 267–72.

Your physician should know that rational combinations of drugs with different and complementary modes of action need to be considered. Research into the pharmacology of various classes of anti-high-blood-pressure drugs has provided extensive information on their mechanisms of action. This knowledge, combined with the results of studies that have clarified mechanisms of blood pressure regulation and prevailing aberrations in different patient populations according to age, race, or other inherent characteristics, has led to rational combinations of drugs from different classes. The two main factors that characterize a rational drug combination are synergistic action, meaning a combined effect that exceeds the additive blood-pressure-lowering effect of each component, and mechanisms of action that offset one another's side effects. In general, the enhanced anti-high-blood-pressure efficacy of synergistic combinations allows lower doses of separate drugs with fewer dose-dependent adverse effects.

Let's look at the various combination therapies in a bit more detail.

ACE Inhibitors and CCBs

The ACE inhibitors and CCBs are one example of a synergistic combination. Certain CCBs stimulate both the renin-angiotensin system and the sympathetic nervous system through vasodilation or expansion of the blood vessels. This causes reflex vasoconstriction, or narrowing of blood vessels, and rapid heartbeat, which may blunt the efficacy of CCBs. ACE inhibitors diminish these reactions and maximize the blood-pressure-lowering effects. ACE inhibitors also counteract the retention of salt and water as well as the edema that CCBs tend to cause. In addition, ACE inhibitors work with CCBs to prevent or reverse diabetic nephropathy as well as adverse effects on the heart.

Angiotensin Inhibitors and Diuretics

The ACE inhibitors and diuretics or ARBs and diuretics are another common example of a synergistic combination. There is a synergistic effect in combining a diuretic and a blocker of the renin-angiotensin system such as an ACE inhibitor or an ARB. In terms of side effects, combination therapy may also be better. For example, diuretics can overstimulate the renin-angiotensin system. Renin is an enzyme that regulates arterial blood pressure. When diuretics overstimulate the renin-angiotensin system, arteries constrict and the body retains water and sodium. The accelerated reaction can also produce lowered potassium and increased uric acid in the blood. The addition of an ACE inhibitor or ARB reduces the overstimulation of the renin-angiotensin system. The result is a maximal lowering of blood pressure!

Captopril and hydrochlorothiazide was an early combination, and is often the reference against which prescriptions of newer ACE inhibitors plus diuretics are compared in several trials over the past few years. The same mechanism is true for ARBs plus various diuretics. An added advantage of these combinations is that the ACE inhibitor or ARB tends to offset not only the compensatory hormonal reactions, but also what are known as dysmetabolic effects of thiazide drugs such as insulin resistance, decreased potassium, and high levels of uric acid in the blood. Furthermore, the addition of a diuretic to either of these angiotensin inhibitors or blockers permits control of blood pressure for patients. For example, some groups with high blood pressure may exhibit resistance to the angiotensin-inhibiting drugs. However, these persons can still benefit from the long-term, end-organ protection of angiotensin inhibition that is widely believed to offer benefits beyond lowered blood pressure.

Beta-Blockers and CCBs

Beta-blockers combined with CCBs may complement each other in their effects. In addition, they minimize or suppress each other's adverse effects. Beta-blockers suppress the stimulation of the renin-angiotensin and sympathetic nervous systems caused by the vasodilatory or blood vessel relaxant effects of CCBs. In return, the CCBs inhibit the tightening of the blood vessels some beta-blockers cause.

Diuretics and Beta-Blockers

Diuretics and beta-blockers have additive blood-pressure-lowering effects but may also interact to accentuate each other's adverse effects, such as sexual dysfunction and accelerated onset of glucose intolerance. In lower doses, however, the intensity and the likelihood of side effects drop. An example of a common fixed low-dose combination is bisoprolol and hydrochlorothiazide. Medical literature reports several such combinations, including fixed three-drug combinations.

A Word about Fixed-Drug Combinations

Fixed-drug combinations attack the blood pressure via two or more mechanisms that, as I mentioned, use lower doses to achieve an effect greater than what each drug could accomplish alone. In fact, these combinations may be more appealing to patients with high blood pressure. A busy patient who wants to bring down blood pressure with fewer doctor visits may be more satisfied if they start anti-high-blood-pressure therapy with a low-dose two-drug combination. For a high-risk patient with severe or dangerously high blood pressure, especially a patient who also has compromised kidney function, diabetes, and elevated risk of heart attack, starting out with fixed-dose combination therapy of three or more drugs at higher doses may help that patient attain a safe blood pressure more rapidly.

For patients that need flexible dosing, several of the combinations listed in Table 7.3 are available in multiple-dose combinations regarding diuretics. However, caution needs to be used with multiple doses. It is often difficult to maximize the dosage of one component such as an ACE inhibitor or an ARB when desired without maximizing a CCB or diuretic. Increasing the dose of the second drug may be undesirable because of the unwelcome possibility of adverse effects. The physician could switch to separate prescriptions. However, the patient may find this upsetting or confusing, and may not maintain the drug regimen. Therefore, many practitioners like to start out with separate drugs that are gradually increased to achieve the target blood pressure and then switch the patient to a fixed combination for chronic maintenance.

Practitioners also switch to fixed combinations because of the eventuality of an adverse reaction, because the side effects from some combinations are easy to detect, such as coughing caused by a combination that contains an ACE inhibitor. However, if a patient starts out with a combination therapy and develops an allergic reaction or digestive problems, the doctor cannot figure out which component is the culprit and thus discards the whole therapy. This phenomenon occurs infrequently, and many physicians prefer fixed combinations to begin medication therapy. As you can see, this can get very complex!

Combinations to Avoid

Some combinations are undesirable or inappropriate. This may be because the combination of drugs has little additional effect on lowering blood pressure than each component alone, such as a CCB plus a diuretic. Worse, the adverse effects of the combined drugs might be additive to the point of becoming dangerous. For example, the diuretic verapamil and a beta-blocker can lead to excessive increased heartbeat and reduced heart contractions.

No matter which combination a physician considers, the choice of an optimal combination therapy comes down to a physician's judgment call. The physician has to weigh blood pressure factors such as age, ethnicity, and diet as well as conditions that coexist with high blood pressure such as heart disease, diabetes, gout, and obesity.

Some believe that future research may develop a "polypill," or a cocktail that features a fixed combination of agents that work on various components of metabolic syndrome as well as other coexisting common high blood pressure risk factors. This polypill combo would treat both high-risk patients with conditions requiring polypharmacy, or more than one drug, and healthy, asymptomatic individuals. It would also include drugs other than anti-high-blood-pressure drugs. The polypill of the future might combine an ACE inhibitor, a beta-blocker, a diuretic, a statin, low-dose aspirin, and so on. The single pill would permit control of several blood and metabolic aberrations.

Regardless of the combinations available and what type of drug therapy your doctor prescribes, it's important in all cases to take medicine correctly and treat it with respect to keep blood pressure under control.

General Guidelines for Taking Blood Pressure Medication

Ultimately, appropriate use of blood pressure medication, where absolutely necessary, saves thousands and likely millions of lives, as well as thousands of dollars in unnecessary procedures! If you need to take your medication to lower your blood pressure, it's important to be consistent and diligent. Diet, exercise, and the regular routines of life can sometimes overload our mental computers. It's easy to skip a day or two of vital medication without even thinking about it. But forgetting to take blood pressure medication can have disastrous consequences. A few missed doses could be fatal.

TAKE is an acronym to help people remember to take prescribed blood pressure drugs.

Time

As your doctor will tell you to do with most drugs, you need to take your blood pressure medications at the same time every day. Try to associate taking the medicine with something else that you do regularly at that time of the day, such as eating breakfast. Many medications usually are taken with food.

Automatic

Make it easy to take your medication. I certainly recommend a small pill box with the days of the week to help with organization. You can buy these containers at Wal-Mart and most drugstores. In fact, everyone (including those that don't take blood pressure medications) should have a pill box in the kitchen. We all should be taking certain vitamin supplements daily. Also, in extreme cases you can use your computer or PDA to set up a customized reminder system. Most people will not need a calendar reminder or Post-it notes all over the house. Taking pills should be as much a part of daily life as brushing your teeth rather than an added burden.

Keep Refilling

With blood pressure medication, especially, always remember to refill your prescription. Form the habit of getting a refill when you have at least a week's supply left in the bottle. Please don't wait until the bottle is empty! What if you are unable to leave the house due to inclement weather or it's a holiday on the day that you actually need the new prescription? Each time you pick up a refill, make a note on your calendar to order and pick up the next refill one week before the medicine is due to run out. However, don't refill too early, as your insurance will typically not pay for the refill.

Fortunately, automated refill services at drugstore chains as well as at Target and Wal-Mart make ordering refills easy. You can also refill your prescriptions online through your pharmacy of choice or services such as Merck-Medco.com.

Emotional Support

Of course, with any healthy habit, it is always important to have a good support system of family and friends. If you have friends and/or family members who also take medication, help remind each other. You do a lot of good for each other medically, and this is a great way to stay in touch. Think of them as part of your medical team, and you get the added boost from being a part of their team.

Finally, know the limitations of your blood pressure medication.

Blood Pressure Medication: An Aid, Not a Cure

One of the most frequent misconceptions about blood pressure medications is that they actually cure high blood pressure. It is true that if someone makes significant lifestyle changes (e.g., diet and exercise), that person may not need medication for high blood pressure anymore.

If you have been on medication for several years and your blood pressure remains normal, it's likely that you'll be able to reduce the dose of medication. In certain cases, medications can be stopped completely. Amazingly, however, at least 50 percent of people with normal blood pressure whose medications were stopped by their physician are still able to stay off medications after one year.

A doctor is the only one who should make the determination that you can "step down" or stop blood pressure drug therapy. *Never just stop taking your medication because you think you feel better!* Stopping your medication without consulting your doctor is risky and could be disastrous, especially with certain kinds of blood pressure medications.

When you do stop taking blood pressure medications, remember that lifestyle modifications will be as important as ever to keep you feeling good.

Other Medication Considerations

People stop taking medication for what they believe are good reasons. The most common is the fear of side effects. It is important to remember that all medications have side effects. It is very important to discuss any potential side effects with your doctor. If no side effects are mentioned, ask about any the doctor may know of. Knowing on the front end may prevent you from stopping medication. Always be open with your health care provider if there is an uncomfortable side effect.

Certainly the ever-spiraling costs of medication and the health insurance maze are additional obstacles for some people who need blood pressure medication. This is why I frequently am asked about brand-name quality versus generic medication. The answer to this question is not a simple yes or no. This answer can depend on the individual. When all other things are equal, sometimes cost prevents someone from getting medication that is needed. If you don't have health insurance or if your provider won't cover certain medications, the cost can be prohibitive. In this case, generic certainly has its advantages.

Whether you choose brand name or generic medication, you need to know whether the medication is effective. Doctors like patients to follow up to assess medications. Sometimes this interval may be every six weeks, every three months, every six months, or once a year. It is very important that doctors determine this on an individual basis. When a person's blood pressure is not where it should be, most doctors ask the patient to return at much shorter intervals, such as in one month. Weekly visits for dose checking are too frequent in most cases, because most popular high blood pressure agents have long serum elimination half-lives. Once-daily anti-high-blood-pressure agents require a few days of administration before achieving a reasonable blood level. Achieving a stable effective level may take twice as long. After the normal blood pressure target is achieved, the visits may be spaced less frequently.

There's one last consideration when you're taking medication. Although, generally, lower blood pressure is better, some caution must also be used with age. Medication therapy, especially combination therapies, could cause an otherwise healthy person to have trouble with maintaining balance and staying alert, let alone a person who already has health issues such as diabetes and cardiovascular problems. As the population ages, doctors and patients need to talk about how to compensate for the effects medication can have on an aging body. If a patient is able to handle separate drug prescriptions and to follow a blood pressure medication regimen, the attending physician can switch a fixed-drug combination therapy to separate prescriptions.

Lou's Story

At 35, "Lou" never thought he'd get high blood pressure, but he developed it after years of high stress from his job as a police officer and his obligation to care for his aging parents, both of whom had heart problems and diabetes. His mother took combination drug therapy but, as she aged, found her alertness and balance reduced. She struggled with the side effects and frequently relied on Lou and his father for help. Lou's father was in poor physical condition himself, so Lou's obligation increased, as did his daily stress. Lou was only slightly overweight and extremely active, but high blood pressure still hit him hard. He was a heavy drinker and smoker before his department insisted he get tested for heart disease.

Lou's doctor prescribed a diuretic to help with volume. Lou had been taking potassium supplements, but "phased them out" on his own. He tried to follow his doctor's advice. He quit smoking and reduced his alcohol intake. However, because of his erratic schedule, he didn't always take his medicine when he was directed. Lou was also self-conscious about telling anyone he took medication. His precinct was a particularly rough-and-tumble one. People looked to Lou to be the strong one who could handle any situation. Some cops considered taking medication a weakness. Lou didn't have anyone to support and help him.

In the meantime, his mother died before she could switch to a new combination drug therapy. Shortly after Lou's mother's death, his father died of grief. Lou had a nonfatal heart attack and his department put him on disability leave. Now Lou was afraid for his life. He took his medication more seriously. His doctor ordered once-a-week medication checks. However, police officer benefits were slashed due to the economy, and Lou found himself unable to afford the brand-name medication he had previously taken. His doctor approved a switch to a generic prescription, and Lou was able to afford the medicine he needed. Lou also took the time to make a schedule that helped him take his medication at breakfast time every day without fail.

Six months later, Lou got a thorough exam from his police department and from his doctor. He passed with flying colors, and the department cleared Lou to return to active duty. Lou still takes care of himself and carries a plastic container for his medication so he doesn't skip a dose when he's on a stakeout. Everyone now knows about Lou's medication, and Lou has discovered he is not the only one in his squad with high blood pressure. Lou's partner and his friends in the department remind him to take his medication. He has remained smoke-free for several months. He has not had another heart attack, and his latest blood pressure exam showed numbers in the normal range. Lou's doctor has monitored him and recently switched him to another diuretic after previous side effects interfered with Lou's normal routine.

Now Lou has been able to discontinue his medication. He keeps up with information about future therapies and has also volunteered for some alternative medicine studies to help further research for others.

A Final Word

I sincerely wish the same success for any of you. If you are taking high blood pressure medication, I hope you may achieve normal blood pressure with diet and exercise—it is certainly possible, as you can see!

A question I'm frequently asked is, "Can I cure high blood pressure with alternative medicine? Is there something better than medication in the future?" I know that there is a wealth of information on alternative and speculative health out there. I'll devote the next chapter to nonpharmaceutical, nondrug alternative, and future therapies.

Chapter 7

ALTERNATIVE APPROACHES TO MEDICATION

WHEN I GIVE TALKS about high blood pressure, I'm often asked about alternative medicine. My answer is always that in general, alternative medicine is neither totally good nor completely harmful. This question is too general to answer, as there are many products and therapies currently being marketed as "alternative," and in particular for treating heart disease and high blood pressure. Products or therapies you most likely have heard about include:

- Hawthorn
- Qigong exercises/yoga
- Ephedra
- Coenzyme Q10 (CoQ10)
- Green tea
- Dark chocolate

I can't make the blanket statement that all alternative therapies are effective, but that does not mean that I am against trying some of these products or therapies, at least those that don't appear to be harmful. To be honest, there are many therapies out there that simply have not been studied enough to determine if they are effective.

People with high blood pressure that seek out alternative therapies do so for various reasons, but most often, these people are, like me, interested in optimum health—not just scraping by on health! This type of consumer-patient wants to feel good while getting healthy. Of course, there is a group of people who choose alternative therapies after a negative experience with Westernized medicine. When both groups of people ask me about complementary alternative medicine (CAM), they wonder which of the many claims out there are true. Learning about alternative medicine often involves sifting through much misinformation and many conflicting opinions.

Unfortunately, many doctors discourage discussion about CAM, and patients tend not to mention whatever complementary therapies they are using. This silence and secrecy creates a bigger dilemma, since untested (and often unregulated) substances or therapies could hinder patients' treatment. Also, alternative therapies could conflict with whatever treatment a physician has prescribed. The other problem is that physicians may not have the slightest idea about complementary and alternative therapies that could be beneficial to patients.

Although I can't fully endorse herbal therapies as of this writing, when I talk to people who have high blood pressure, I always encourage open discussion about the potential benefits and harms of CAM therapies and products that my audience may use. I also know that more and more of my fellow physicians no longer exclude CAM from health practices. Many colleagues suggest the use of herbal remedies, diet, and alternative medicine as natural health solutions for living a healthy life.

Dietary Supplements

Some people reading this may have the idea that herbal and diet remedies involve visiting a hippie farmer with an overgrown vegetable garden and a drying shed. The reality is that herbal and dietary supplements now line the shelves of major store chains and are very much mainstream.

Dietary supplements were defined by the Dietary Supplement Health and Education Act of 1994 as "a product taken orally, and intended to supplement the diet." Dietary supplements include vitamins, minerals, herbs, and other botanicals, amino acids, enzymes, organ tissues, glandulars (probably not a term everyone has heard of), and metabolites. The Food and Drug Administration (FDA) regulates dietary supplements differently than prescription and over-the-counter drugs. For the most part, the FDA does not require dietary supplement manufacturers to prove safety or efficacy.

Although manufacturing practices have typically been less stringent than for prescription drugs, this is changing. One recent change requires manufacturers and distributors of dietary supplements to submit information to the FDA concerning adverse reactions reported to them by the public. This amendment to the process at least helps to address public-safety concerns.

Despite these changes, some of you reading this book still have questions as to which dietary supplements are worthwhile. However, I would argue that diet and exercise modifications, which I have already talked about, qualify as complementary and alternative therapies as well. Furthermore, many other alternative therapies have been shown to be effective, especially when combined with diet and exercise. In Chapter 3, I mentioned the importance of a daily vitamin/mineral supplement, which I would again recommend highly. Please visit my Web site at http://www.shop.youroptimumhealth.net if you would like more info.

There's not enough room in one chapter for a guide to every alternative therapy available today. But I'll try to discuss several of the main ones as well as future therapies that seem promising, and even tackle the hot-button issue of stem cells very briefly. Most therapies can be categorized as good, unproven, or unsafe.

The Good

Omega-3/Fish Oil

You have likely heard about the tremendous heart-health benefits of omega-3 fatty acids that you take in the form of fish oil or flaxseed oil. Most of their popularity stems from the positive impact on bad lipids (fats) such as triglycerides. I've seen some evidence that the two main omega-3 fatty acids, EPA and DHA, may reduce blood pressure in people with mild high blood pressure. Again, these results haven't been confirmed, but with the known proven, positive effects of omega-3s, you can reasonably try fish oil or flaxseed oil, in liquid or capsule supplements, with no downside. Please refer to my Web site, http://www.shop.youroptimumhealth.net, for more information.

Yoga, Qigong, and T'ai Chi

Stress reduction is one of the most important ways to lower your blood pressure. We'll talk more in Chapter 8 about the tremendous role that stress plays in high blood pressure. Ancient relaxation methods that include controlled breathing and gentle physical activity, such as yoga, qigong, and t'ai chi, are beneficial.

Most everyone is familiar with yoga. Yoga satisfies criteria for physical activity and can actually help improve fitness level. The conscious breathing practiced in yoga reduces stress, and the relaxation of the muscular system brought about by yoga increases blood flow, especially blood flow to the brain and heart, through improved circulation throughout the body.

Specific yoga poses (known as asanas) that lower blood pressure include a classic meditative sitting pose (sukhasana), the cat pose (bidalasana), half spinal twist (ardha matsayendrasana), as well as double leg raises and the stand spread-leg forward fold. In addition, specific conscious breathing exercises such as Uijayi Pranayama may affect certain parts of the body, which could help reduce blood pressure.

T'ai chi chuan, an ancient balance and flexibility practice, is becoming more and more popular in the United States, and has long been thought especially beneficial for elderly people who are sedentary and may benefit from its gentle, gradual movements. Systolic blood pressure after t'ai chi exercises decreases in high blood pressure patients at approximately the same rate as after moderate-intensity aerobic exercise. As with yoga, the emphasis on conscious breathing and the muscular relaxation reduces stress, enhances blood flow to the brain, and improves the circulatory system. Slow, measured breathing associated with t'ai chi helps reduce oxygen levels and therefore the demand for oxygen.

Qigong is likely known least in the western hemisphere. However, the possible blood-pressure-lowering benefits of qigong (also known as chi kung) are comparable to those enjoyed by yoga and t'ai chi chuan practitioners. Qigong includes a combination of isometric exercise (when muscular contractions occur without movement of the body parts being worked), isotonic exercises (when a contracting muscle shortens against a constant load, as when lifting a weight), aerobic conditioning, meditation, and relaxation. All of these exercises may, of course, guard against metabolic syndrome and aid weight control.

Studies conducted at our health facilities have indicated that people with mild high blood pressure who practiced these healing techniques daily for two to three months experienced significant decreases in their blood pressure, had lower levels of stress hormones, and were less anxious. Although there is still a need for larger studies to confirm these potential effects, the fact that there is very minimal to no potential for harm in these strategies makes them attractive to consider. Certain populations, such as elderly and sedentary patients or people with limited mobility, need evaluation by a doctor before starting any type of physical activity program.

Bath Therapy (Balneotherapy)

Herbal baths may sound strange, but many bubble baths or bath soak products already use herbs such as rosemary or mint. Bath therapy has become quite popular. The umbrella term *balneotherapy* refers to mineral spa baths and various spa water treatments involving either drinking or bathing in therapeutic waters. Many physicians believe bathing may be therapeutic for selected medical conditions. Many types of balneotherapy have special means by which they increase or modify their influence; for example, "aromatic" or "medicated" baths. In these baths, substances are mixed to exert a special influence on the circulation and nerves. Popular substances used include pine needle and fir wood oil, an alcoholic extract "tincture," or aromatic herbs such as chamomile or thyme. In my experience, the relaxation and stress reduction associated with these baths play the largest role in the lowering of blood pressure that patients report after enjoying one of these health-spa experiences.

Massage

Everyone likes massage, regardless of any health benefits. One way to help stave off high blood pressure is massage therapy. A number of long-term studies have shown that a consistent massage program can decrease diastolic and systolic blood pressure and decrease cortisol or stress hormone levels, which are also reduced in relaxation techniques such as yoga, t'ai chi, and qigong. Massage lowers anxiety and hostility, which are linked to high blood pressure. The ultimate goal of massage therapy is a pain-free and relaxing lifestyle. Controlling blood pressure is just one of the added benefits of massage therapy.

Amino Acids

Specific herbs and foods can help lower blood pressure. Amino acids, which are not related to fatty acids, build the proteins in our bodies. The amino acid supplements L-arginine and L-taurine may also result in lower blood pressure with generally few side effects. These amino acids usually work in my experience, but I always advise people that amino acids may be less effective depending on individual circumstances. I always refer people to a registered dietitian. Also, amino acids in excess may be detrimental, as with many good things.

Stevia

Outside of herbal remedies, some foods may have more magic in them than meets the eye and may also be considered alternative and complementary. Stevia is a natural sweetener on the market that doesn't get quite as much attention as, say, aspartame-based sweeteners, although maybe it should, since it's said to have up to 300 times the sweetness of sugar. Stevia, which comes from the South American plant stevia rebaudiana, may also be a rich source of antioxidants, specifically quercetin, apigenin, and kaempferol, which protect against DNA damage and cancer.

Stevia is now available in the United States. Truvia is a brand name that I would recommend. For more information, please visit my Web site at http://www.shop.youroptimumhealth.net.

As you may have guessed, I believe much more research is necessary to further explore the potential health benefits of stevia, but researchers express excitement about the potential. Stevia may aid in blood pressure control, not by direct effects but by the indirect effect of controlling excess calories and obesity. The exception is if patients are taking certain calcium channel blockers (CCBs), since stevia can increase the potency of the drug by acting as another calcium antagonist.

Dark Chocolate

There is now good news for chocolate lovers who thought their addiction to chocolate had them doomed. Eating a small amount of dark chocolate every day may slightly lower blood pressure without increasing weight or presenting other health risks. This effect is due largely to the amounts of cocoa polyphenols, a type of antioxidant. However, consuming large amounts of cocoa actually does lead to higher intakes of sugar, fat, and calories, and the long-term outcomes of chocolate consumption are still being explored. Don't be too quick to believe that you need chocolate with every meal now because it is shown to have benefits—remember moderation!

Green Tea

Moving away from chocolate, some healthy beverages are not quite as calorie dense as chocolate. Most of you have probably heard of green tea, which has been used for thousands of years in China and is now popular in the United States. You may have seen the countless preparations, including green tea cookies, ice cream, and soda, available at the grocery and specialty food stores. There does seem to be very positive evidence that green tea reduces blood pressure (or I wouldn't be mentioning it) by repressing the enzyme angiotensin II, which you remember from the last chapter. In essence, green tea acts as an ACE inhibitor. The antioxidant EGCG gives green tea its bite and aids blood health. In addition, green tea may help the heart by lowering total cholesterol levels and improving the ratio of good HDL cholesterol to bad LDL cholesterol. Besides having positive effects on cholesterol, green tea may also inhibit the abnormal formation of blood clots. Green tea may even aid the weight loss that is so crucial in lowering blood pressure!

I recommend further study on green tea, since high doses of it normally cause blood vessels to constrict. Green tea contains a third of the caffeine in coffee, but high doses of green tea extract can have a cumulative effect that increases blood pressure.

Grape Juice/Resveratrol

I've already discussed red wine, but those who don't drink alcohol can still benefit. Grape juice has been demonstrated in limited study to improve the flexibility of your arteries and thus facilitate blood flow, therefore reducing blood pressure. Resveratrol, which I talked about in the red wine section, is found in grape compounds in general and combats heart disease, degenerative nerve disease, and other ailments. However, even unsweetened grape juice has some glucose, and I repeat my familiar refrain about moderation. Grape juice, like the treatments and therapies in this section, is something I can advocate for high blood pressure patients without much reservation.

The Unproven

Several herbal and physical therapies also seem to benefit blood pressure. Some supplements are thought to aid in lowering blood pressure, but the jury is still out.

Coenzyme Q10

Coenzyme Q10 (CoQ10), which is necessary for the functioning of body cells, appears to produce small reductions in systolic and diastolic blood pressure. CoQ10 is thought to reduce blood pressure by a different mechanism than most prescription medications. Taking CoQ10 supplements boosts the body's natural supply of the enzyme that decreases with age and is low in patients with heart disease.

It's not clear whether low CoQ10 is a cause of high blood pressure. I haven't found definitive evidence of the long-term efficiency of CoQ10 supplements in lowering high blood pressure and diminishing heart disease, and I would argue that the long-term effects need to be studied. However, the modest drop in systolic and diastolic blood pressure seen after people take CoQ10 supplements is a positive sign, and taking these supplements can't hurt. There have been some reports of side effects when it is taken in conjunction with vigorous exercise, so if you do take CoQ10, you may want to opt for moderate-intensity aerobic exercise.

Hawthorn (Crataegus species)

Hawthorn is readily available in capsule form and may be effective in bringing about positive results for the heart and circulatory system, including blood pressure. Hawthorn, however, is one of the stronger herbal medicines and should therefore always be discussed with a doctor first. Overdose can cause cardiac arrhythmia and dangerously lower blood pressure. Milder side effects include nausea and sedation.

Mud Baths

When I mentioned balneotherapy, some readers probably thought, "Does that mean mud baths?" As a matter of fact, mud bathing is one less-proven aspect of balneotherapy. Mud baths are chiefly prepared from muddy deposits found around springs. They act like a large porridge applied to the surface of the body, and in addition to the influence of the warm or hot bath temperature that can be therapeutic, the mud deposits raise the respiration number and accelerate the pulse by six to twelve beats per minute. Although this type of balneotherapy is thought to be beneficial for fibromyalgia syndrome, gout, and other rheumatic conditions, don't count on mud bathing for better blood pressure control. It may relax you and decrease stress, but any direct effect on blood pressure remains to be seen.

Acupuncture

Some of my colleagues will deny the value of acupuncture. Even though more studies without major weaknesses are needed to determine whether or not acupuncture treats high blood pressure, the truth is that acupuncture can be very effective in the right situation with a reputable acupuncturist whose credentials have been vetted. Acupuncture has been shown to relieve abdominal distention/flatulence, chronic pain, allergic sinusitis, anorexia, anxiety, arthritis, carpal tunnel syndrome, cervical and lumbar spine syndromes, frozen shoulder, headache, muscle spasms, tremors, contractures, nerve pain, plantar fasciitis, premenstrual syndrome, skin disorders, sleep disorders, and sprains.

I know that even though most states require a license to practice acupuncture, education and training standards and requirements for obtaining a license to practice vary from state to state. Because very few medical doctors actually practice acupuncture and are licensed to do so, it is important to find someone qualified. Although a license does not ensure quality of care, it does indicate that the practitioner meets set standards regarding the knowledge and use of acupuncture. That said, you should not put too much stock in an acupuncturist telling you that you have high blood pressure if that acupuncturist does not have substantial medical training. If you have received a diagnosis of high blood pressure from a doctor, you may wish to ask your doctor whether acupuncture might help.

Reflexology

You read the praises of massage as a blood pressure reduction therapy. Reflexology is a specialized massage that applies pressure to the feet and hands with specific thumb, finger, and hand techniques without the use of oil or lotion. The benefits of reflexology primarily have to do with the reduction of stress, since the hands and fingers may interrupt the stress signals. The relaxation produced by reflexology is similar to the effects of body massage. Whether or not reflexology can benefit some conditions and diseases is still under investigation. I believe further scientific study needs to be done in order to come to some definite benefits of reflexology in regard to illness and disease. It is possible that reflexology may be a complement to standard medical care. However, it alone should not be a replacement for medical help. Some say that reflexology actually helps the mechanism of the heart that regulates blood pressure, but this is a stretch and an unverified claim. But I believe reflexology does no harm.

The Unsafe

As I mentioned, the efficacy and safety of many herbal therapies for treating high blood pressure have not been extensively studied. Because of potential health risks associated with the following herbs, you need to consider avoiding them if you are also taking high blood pressure medication. If you are not taking medication, it's wise to use caution when taking the herbs and to monitor any changes in your blood pressure and overall physical well-being:

- **Tetrandrine (Stephania tetrandra)**—Although tetrandrine (used in the treatment of edema) can lower blood pressure, you should avoid tetrandrine if you are taking verapamil. Like stevia, tetrandrine acts as a calcium antagonist and can amplify the effects of verapamil.

Some herbal preparations are harmful to high blood pressure patients. You should avoid the following herbal therapies because they can increase blood pressure. Even one dose could be too much.

- **Yohimbe/yohimbine**—Yohimbine comes from the yohimbe bark of a West African evergreen tree and is used to treat erectile dysfunction and to boost blood pressure in patients with low blood pressure. Athletes have also used it as a weight-loss aid. Large doses of it raise blood pressure to dangerous levels in people with high blood pressure.
- **Licorice**—Taking licorice supplements, drinking licorice tea, or even eating licorice raises blood pressure.
- **Ephedra/ephedrine/má huáng/pseudoephedrine**—Ephedra is on the list not because it's a therapy for blood pressure but because people take it for energy, weight loss, and athletic performance. Ephedra is a form of the active ingredient used in many decongestants and asthma drugs, and has been used in traditional Chinese medicine for 5,000 years for the treatment of asthma and hay fever, as well as for the common cold. It raises heart rate and blood pressure, and is

dangerous for those with high blood pressure, heart disease, or diabetes. It increases heart rate and constricts blood vessels, thereby increasing blood pressure. You may have already read warnings about ephedra in numerous other books and articles. Ephedrine (a derivative of ephedra) was used as an asthma drug until the early 1980s, when doctors stopped prescribing it because of its dangerous effects on the heart and blood pressure. The synthetic form of another ephedra ingredient, pseudoephedrine, is still used in many over-the-counter decongestants, which carry strong warning labels and are meant for only short-term use. Common cold remedies made with pseudoephedrine can be very dangerous in persons with high blood pressure and even apparently healthy young people.

- **Ephedra-related products/guarana/kola nut/yerba mate—** Other products or ingredients have ephedra or relatives of it, though it may not always be obvious. For instance, *Sida cordifolia* (country mallow) supplies ephedra compounds; also "Mormon tea" and "desert tea" are actually types of ephedra. Some manufacturers add other herbs, such as guarana, yerba mate, and kola nut (all high in caffeine) to give extra kick to supplements. Guarana may increase the risk of stroke, bleeding, heart attack, and sudden death. Ephedra is directly associated with increases in heart rate, blood pressure, and potentially harmful changes in glucose and potassium levels. Then a range of products purport to stimulate the thyroid. It's unsafe to take anything that might boost thyroid hormones, and the FDA has cracked down on some of these supplements. Hypothyroidism (too little thyroid hormone) and hyperthyroidism (too much thyroid hormone) can both lead to high blood pressure. Unbelievably, news reports say many doctors are now selling ephedra and other such supplements to patients. If this is recommended to you for weight loss, it should raise many questions. This is a dangerous way to try to shed a few pounds.

- **Bitter orange extract (*Citrus aurantium*)—**Another "herb" to stay away from totally is bitter orange extract, which is derived from the rind of Seville oranges. One of the ingredients is synephrine, which is similar to the potent chemical in ephedra, acts like ephedra, and speeds up calorie burning, but it may also raise blood pressure and heart rate. Bitter orange extract contains methyltyramine, which raises blood pressure.

- **DMAE (Dimethylaminoethanol)**—DMAE is a supplement that was once sold as a prescription drug for treating learning difficulties. However, it was taken off the market because of insufficient evidence that it worked. It is still allowed in supplements, and it is known to raise blood pressure and cause insomnia. Avoid DMAE.

Although I have just touched the surface, with all herbal and nutritional remedies, drug interactions should be considered. I have to admit that I am not familiar with all of the proposed remedies out there, and many are not native to the United States. There are many good references out there to help avoid these interactions if you take certain medications. Recent reports in the literature of cases of excessive or inappropriate use of herbal dietary supplements have led to the term "polyherbacy." At this point there are no recommended daily doses for most experimental herbs, so you use them at your own risk. I may sound like a broken record, but moderation is important if you want to ensure that the cure is not more life-threatening or unpleasant than the disease.

When people hear my stance on various alternative healing methods, the follow-up question is, "Isn't science going to find us a cure in the future, like on *Star Trek*? What if we just change our genes or body chemistry to keep our blood pressure low?"

Future Therapies

The future world of science fiction has its roots in the experimental therapies being studied and developed today. Although we don't have computers that can diagnose and treat you in minutes or even seconds, future advancements in medicine have the potential to get us all closer to our optimum health!

Gene Therapy/Genomics

Years after the completion of the Human Genome Project, researchers continue to express both excitement and skepticism about the near-term applications of genomics in health care and disease prevention.

Some public health scientists view genomics research on high blood pressure as low priority. As we've seen, the major preventable causes of blood pressure are obesity, lack of exercise, tobacco abuse, excess alcohol abuse, and unhealthy diet. However, as I mentioned in Chapter 1, genes can play a role in high blood pressure, along with lifestyle factors. I mentioned that right now you can't do anything about your genes. In the future, this may not be absolutely true.

Gene therapy may ultimately be a means to treat high blood pressure in humans. Scientific research on lab animals funded by the National Institutes of Health has led to the blocking of a protein in the kidneys that triggers high blood pressure and kidney damage. This promising technique may prove to be effective in preventing the progression of high blood pressure.

Nutrigenomics

Nutrigenomics is an area of science that seems very promising in helping individuals understand health risks that may be specifically related to one's own genetic makeup. Nutrigenomics is the study of food and diet and how nutrition interacts with specific genes to increase the risk of different diseases. By identifying various genes that affect heart health, bone health, chronic inflammation, fitness levels, obesity risks, and other components of healthy living, doctors can now tailor recommendations to an individual's unique genetic makeup. Physicians use nutrigenomics to gain insight into your genetic makeup and use that information to guide you in making key lifestyle choices to achieve this potential. This of course includes heart health and the health of the blood vessels. Specific dietary changes can be made to counteract genetic weaknesses, such as the predisposition to high blood pressure.

This prospect is certainly exciting, but the technology is still in early stages and is not widespread. I see it to have extreme importance as we begin to focus more on prevention as opposed to waiting until after the fact! It is still yet to be seen how these dietary changes actually affect health, but it appears very promising.

Stem Cell Questions

Inevitably, I receive questions about the much-debated and exceedingly controversial stem cells as a treatment for high blood pressure.

Adult stem cells have been used to treat diseases including many blood and immune system–related genetic diseases, some cancers, juvenile diabetes, Parkinson's disease, blindness, and spinal cord injuries. The body uses adult stem cells to repair specific cell types when injured. Some stem cells injected with nitric oxide are being used in experimental treatments to repair and protect blood vessels and improve blood flow to bring down high blood pressure. The most promise of this technique lies in curing pulmonary high blood pressure.

The issue becomes sticky when we consider using embryonic stem cells, which can differentiate 220 cell types in the adult body. Some argue that this potential remains for adult stem cells, but it is still under debate among scientists.

Whatever CAM treatments you are considering, future or current therapies, taking the time to educate yourself about your options and alternatives will serve you well in the long run. I wish all members of the medical establishment were open to or at least knowledgeable about CAM.

A Word for Physicians

As demand and need for all of these complementary therapies have increased, so too has the public's expectation that health care professionals be knowledgeable about CAM and prepared to advise patients. In 2000, the National Institutes of Health National Center for Complementary and Alternative Medicine began awarding competitive, five-year educational grants to academic institutions committed to teaching CAM content to health professional students.

This latest development recognizes that the world of preventive, complementary, and alternative medicine has exploded onto the scene! Whether it is advancement in genetics, vaccines, or herbal treatments, science is constantly evolving. It is important that with these changes and discoveries we do not become stubborn in our thinking, but continue to be open-minded. There are, however, some basic principles in medicine that are not changing, and we must also remember this as well.

This chapter highlights potential alternative strategies to possibly augment blood pressure disease management needs. The use of CAM may offer some patients and doctors an opportunity to enhance efforts to curtail the increasing prevalence of hypertension in our country. Those in public health could help facilitate such an approach and a launch pad for further research and practice in CAM and the management of high blood pressure as we move further into the twenty-first century.

When people have reliable alternatives, and when we as doctors are willing to work with high blood pressure patients to improve treatment methods, the result is less worry and anxiety, and therefore stress, for people with high blood pressure. This dovetails well with my final ideas for bringing down high blood pressure: de-stressing to improve your life.

Chapter 8

DE-STRESSING TO PROLONG YOUR LIFE

HAVE YOU EVER BEEN in the checkout line at the grocery store and gotten a bit "hot under the collar" because the person three carts ahead has had a problem with the credit card transaction and a manager has been called to resolve the situation?

Or have you ever been late for an appointment and missed your exit on the freeway because the drivers in the right lane didn't make room for you?

Have you ever suppressed anger and resentment because a coworker or your boss piles too much criticism and work on you, or when your spouse or children take you for granted and don't acknowledge that you have needs?

It seems like an eternity in that grocery store situation when you're waiting for the manager to arrive from the receiving area in the rear of the store. You're already running through the endless list of things you have to do and you're getting more anxious by the second. Similarly, on the freeway, you're starting to feel "road rage" because you're already late and going to the next exit will add another 10 minutes to your arrival time. You panic, you feel guilty, and you worry. At work and at home, you won't express your emotions for fear of jeopardizing your job or causing domestic strife.

Whether you realize it or not, in the above situations that nearly everyone has experienced, you also boost your blood pressure as much as if you had smoked a pack of cigarettes or eaten a supersize portion of French fries. Those stressful emotions and thoughts travel right to your heart and cause your blood vessels to constrict. These situations may actually be dangerous to your own health.

However, if you ever feel like you are just going to explode because the walls of the world are closing in on you at one time, you are not alone in your responses to stress. A conservative estimate suggests that greater than 60 percent of working people are affected negatively by stress. However, thanks to the techniques and suggestions I discuss in this chapter, they have learned to manage if not eliminate stress, and you can do it too. Stress is certainly everywhere and can be difficult to avoid in today's society, but if you can reduce stress, you have done your health a world of good!

The Direct Line from Stress to High Blood Pressure

Whenever you feel threatened by a long line, a deadline, or an accident, the hormone called adrenaline increases dramatically in your bloodstream. Adrenaline is life-saving in a crisis, and as you have probably read, it aided our prehistoric ancestors to survive in harsh environments. We have progressed from fighting saber-toothed tigers to struggling against heavy traffic and computer viruses. Often when our bodies experience what is commonly referred to as the fight-or-flight response, the likelihood of physical danger is not as great as in our ancestors' time, unless you are in a war zone. However, the biochemistry remains the same as it was millions of years ago.

When you are afraid or upset, nerve impulses in your brain shout "red alert" to the adrenal glands that are located at the upper end of the kidneys. The adrenal glands release a flood of adrenaline into the bloodstream and kick the bodily processes into high gear. Your heart rate increases as your heart pounds, and the volume of blood pumped also increases. Your blood vessels constrict. Adrenaline also causes the release of extra glucose (sugar) to the muscles, creating a battle rush. Interestingly, smoking cigarettes produces the same effect, although, again, repeated stress and adrenaline release may be more toxic in the long run. Once the threat, or perceived threat, has passed, adrenaline disappears. This allows the heartbeat and blood pressure to return to normal levels.

During the stress response, somewhere in the neighborhood of 1,500 biochemical reactions occur in the body. Neurotransmitters are activated, hormones are released, and nutrients are metabolized. The cardiovascular system accelerates its function, while other systems such as the digestive system slow down their operations in response to stress. Unfortunately, the by-products of the stress response continue to circulate in the body and have the potential to create physical illness. We now know that stress is one of the important factors in heart disease and GERD (gastroesophageal reflux disease), both very common medical conditions in the United States. In addition, people use unhealthy behaviors to cope with stress, specifically overeating, smoking, and abusing alcohol, which are directly related to high blood pressure.

In manifold ways, stress can significantly compromise the quality of life for millions and millions of Americans, for whom daily stresses have become the norm. Studies undertaken at medical institutions confirm through research the role of emotions in heart disease, high blood pressure, and other conditions. The anger and hostility that many of us repress contribute to the hidden tension and anxiety that drives up blood pressure and weakens immune system function.

Short-term links between stress/repressed emotions and blood pressure create long-term risks. Even temporary spikes in blood pressure caused by stress and/or anger can cause damage to major organs if those spikes occur often enough. These temporary shocks to the system can damage your blood vessels, heart, and kidneys in the same way that persistent high blood pressure does. Possible links between long-term stress and high blood pressure exist. After you've been diagnosed with high blood pressure, you can make a lasting difference in your cardiovascular health by understanding those connections. However, you can act before it's too late!

Lorenzo's Story

The golden years were not as Lorenzo had dreamed they would be. After retirement, he didn't know what to do with the rest of his life. Long-divorced, he dated women that he met online and he traveled. He threw himself into playing golf and occasionally volunteering at the local homeless shelter. But none of his dates went anywhere because he was still attached to his ex-wife. Even the allure of activity faded, and he spent more and more time alone playing computer games or watching television to avoid loneliness. He gained at least 40 pounds in what seemed like no time at all and had abdominal fat. He began drinking, at first in the evening, then throughout the day. His sleep patterns became disturbed, and he either stayed awake for days or slept most of the day, which caused him to suffer alone at night when he needed to sleep the most.

One day Lorenzo was in line at the dry cleaner's, and the woman ahead of him spent what seemed like an hour, even though it was only 10 minutes, giving detailed instructions on how she wanted her sheets laundered. Lorenzo lost his temper and screamed at complete strangers as well as the owner of the shop, with whom he had developed a friendly relationship. The young clerk, who was new on the job, burst into tears. The owner offered Lorenzo a complimentary suit-pressing to get him to calm down, but Lorenzo thought of how he didn't need a suit and got more upset. His chest felt tight, and he got so dizzy he went to his car and lay in the backseat for an hour until the security guard for the shopping center checked on him. The guard told him he needed to "chill out."

Lorenzo's friends called him because word had gotten out about the incident, and people recalled that Lorenzo had made several scenes in public lately when he felt inconvenienced. At first Lorenzo felt angry— people treated him with disrespect in public. He got so upset he nearly collapsed. Alarms went off in his head and he suddenly saw himself as an angry, bitter old man. He went to our health facility the next morning.

The doctor knew that years ago Lorenzo had been told he had high blood pressure. Lorenzo rejected pills and medication. While he was still active and important, Lorenzo was able to keep himself healthy and balanced and to lower his blood pressure without drugs. Now that Lorenzo was under stress, his blood pressure had skyrocketed to 160/100, far above the recommended level!

Lorenzo was confused. He was retired. How could he have stress? The doctor referred him to a counselor at our facility who helped him understand that his frustration at no longer doing what he'd done most of his life, his repressed anger and guilt over the breakup of his marriage, and the resentment toward the people who'd once mistreated him created internal stress. Every time those old feelings reawakened when he felt he was being taken advantage of, he put a strain on his blood vessels, his heart, and his immune system, and he didn't even know he was silently destroying himself. Lorenzo had once been a devout Catholic. He remembered forgotten Christian teachings about trusting in the Divine and God, about mastering one's emotions, and about forgiveness and compassion.

He began to take stock of his life. He let go of his past emotional baggage. He called his ex-wife and developed an amicable relationship with her. He reconnected with his children, from whom he'd been estranged. He learned to enjoy doing nothing. Spending an hour a day in meditation and prayer helped him be calm and still inside. He understood that he needn't identify himself with his career.

Doctors and counselors kept watch on Lorenzo in the months to come. He put himself on a strict diet and exercise regimen. He now golfs five days a week, and recently started aerobic exercise classes. He has joined Alcoholics Anonymous and stopped drinking. He has resumed regular sleep patterns and gets six to seven hours of restful sleep.

Lorenzo has volunteered for local charitable causes and now travels more. He apologized to the dry cleaner as well as others he yelled at previously, and has become the genial fellow everyone knew. He has lost much of the weight he gained.

Most importantly, his blood pressure has dropped to 125/80, and he now feels hopeful and optimistic about life for the first time in years.

The Right Stress Relievers and Nature's Cure

As you saw in Lorenzo's history, people often don't do anything about anger, stress, or anxiety until one day they "explode" in anger over minor inconveniences. This can take the form of arguing in public, or as we have seen in far too many shooting incidents and traffic accidents, workplace or road rage. Because of common decency, most people will never open fire and kill innocent people just because of a bad day or a string of bad days. The majority of us, as evidenced by our rampant illnesses and obesity, will instead, in a sense, attack ourselves. We survive one situation and resolve to keep our cool or just "don't worry, be happy." However, we forget to prevent our destructive responses to stress when we're confronted with the next unpleasant situation in our lives.

The good news is that we can modify stress and prevent a negative cycle from recurring, as Lorenzo's example proves. His remedies for anxiety illustrate my belief that it's important to choose the right remedies for stress, not just those stress relievers that offer a quick fix. For example, it's probably not a good idea to routinely have a cold beer or two after work. One or two beers can easily turn into five. In Lorenzo's case, he thought that he didn't have any need to limit his alcohol intake since he no longer had work or family responsibilities, but alcohol can become a problem no matter what your circumstances are. The same holds true for food, especially when combined with a sedentary lifestyle, as we've seen. Try not to be an emotional eater.

In contrast, exercise is nature's cure for stress. It is the most practical intervention ever devised—it is as effective as a visit to a spa (which not everyone may be able to afford in terms of money and/or time). I will probably begin to sound like a CD on endless repeat when it comes to my beliefs about physical activity. I'm not alone, however. Many medical studies support the link between stress relief and exercise.

How does fitness eliminate tension and anxiety? Regular exercise removes the by-products of the stress response that we have mentioned. Dancing, jogging, kickboxing, and swimming provide the opportunity to simulate the fighting or running dictated by the aforementioned fight-or-flight phenomenon and to counteract adrenaline, provided you are not engaging in extreme sports enjoyed by "adrenaline junkies." As such, regular exercise allows the body to return to normal function (also known as homeostasis) faster and reduce the physical impact of psychosocial stress.

More specifically, exercise activates certain beneficial chemical responses in the brain and body. A substantial body of studies on exercise and stress shows that catecholamines, including the well-known beta-endorphins, increase in the blood during physical activity of 20 minutes or more. Beta-endorphins are chemically similar to opiate compounds, and like opiates, provide a safe pain-relieving or analgesic effect. In a sense, exercise produces a euphoria similar to morphine, but eminently safer. This is where we get the term "runner's high." The positive mood changes associated with frequent exercise are so significant, some have suggested that it is a very effective treatment for clinical depression, and often a good alternative to either psychotherapy or antidepressant drugs.

Ironically, many people with chronic stress complain that they seldom have time to exercise, a fallacy I've addressed before. Oddly, surveys of CEOs of Fortune 500 companies indicate that these high-powered executives exercise on a regular basis. They believe they have the time, and so they are able to create time to exercise. I won't rehash all the suggestions about working exercise into your life that you've previously read. I will simply make an appeal for you to try exercise. Or rather, I'll use the commonly heard words of young women going through some difficult life changes and weight gain regarding exercise and stress: "I think my goals in my career and life will work out better this time around now that I'm getting fit. I didn't always make time for exercise and I'd get completely burned out. Stress was ruining my life, but I feel better now that I'm exercising. I'm sleeping better and I have more energy."

And Speaking of Sleep . . .

Did you know that lack of sleep has been linked to high blood pressure? Sleep is often the first thing we neglect when we're under stress, and the rising numbers of overtired Americans show that we are a habitually stressed-out and sleepless nation. Some high achievers can operate at peak efficiency on four or five hours of sleep, as Bill Clinton reportedly did when he occupied the White House, but most adults need seven to eight hours to be fully functional. This is doubly true if you have high blood pressure. And even though one may function without optimal sleep, this doesn't mean all is well.

The American Heart Association has recently reported a study that finds that if you're middle aged and sleep five hours or less a night, you may be increasing your risk of developing high blood pressure. The study's researchers found that nearly 25 percent of people ages 32 to 59 who slept for five or fewer hours a night were significantly more likely to develop high blood pressure. The study's subjects who slept the recommended seven or eight hours were less than half as likely to be diagnosed with high blood pressure. This finding took into account all the other factors that can contribute to high blood pressure I have previously discussed.

Women especially may be at risk, according to a 2007 study in the journal *Hypertension*. Women who slept five hours or less per night and women who slept six hours per night were at significantly greater risk to develop high blood pressure than women who enjoyed a solid seven hours. However, studies across the board show that long-term sleep deprivation seems to increase susceptibility to high blood pressure.

You might ask why sleeplessness raises your blood pressure. For one thing, sleep deprivation causes you to experience stress and irritability, which, as we've seen, create damaging spikes in high blood pressure. More importantly, sleep permits the heart to slow down, which means that blood pressure drops, for a significant part of your daily cycle. However, people who sleep for only short durations raise their average 24-hour blood pressure and heart rate. As you have learned, this rise in heart rate and blood pressure causes an elevated pressure in the blood vessels. In addition, sleep deprivation has been shown previously to increase appetite and compromise insulin sensitivity, which brings about diabetes associated with high blood pressure. Lack of sleep also increases the production of the stress hormone cortisol. People who sleep too little (and interestingly, people who sleep too much) are more likely to be overweight, another risk factor for high blood pressure.

I'll resist the temptation to repeat any of the tips for getting a good night's sleep. A reputable local sleep center has many excellent resources to help you get a better night's rest. I also know that many of you who are reading this book may suffer from obstructive sleep apnea, in which millions of Americans do not breathe when they sleep, or other sleep disorders.

I certainly agree with expert pulmonologists and neurologists who warn that high blood pressure is associated with obstructive sleep apnea as well as other sleep disorders. Sleep apnea is usually treated through a type of oxygen mask called a CPAP that patients wear at night to help facilitate breathing while sleeping. If you have a sleep disorder or think you have a sleep disorder, I encourage you to get treatment. You'll likely lower your high blood pressure and improve your heart health!

Getting enough sleep is a simple step, but it is one that too often gets overlooked. This next suggestion, however, may be the most important of all.

Increase Your Faith, Decrease Your Worries

The subject of one's religion is often a hot-button issue, since religion and spirituality are deeply personal. However, I believe not introducing the topic of faith may do more damage to a patient's mental, emotional, and physical well-being.

Spirituality, prayer, and worship can help relieve the tension and anxiety we often feel in modern life, and there is certainly truth to being able to "pray one's way to great health." While many of us take the wonderful benefits of genuine faith for granted, a growing body of medical evidence shows that prayer and spirituality assist in healing, even from life-threatening conditions and illnesses. Research has shown the effect of prayer on patients undergoing heart procedures to be very positive and with significantly fewer side effects. I have observed that a patient's individual belief is often proof enough for that individual, and what matters in the healing process is that patient's religious belief.

A medical facility that provides faith-based compassionate medical care is certainly wonderful. I am up-front about my religion with the people who read this book and the people who ask me for answers. I tell them I believe that having faith in God does improve health. It certainly provides a sense of peace that helps people cope with stress.

Many women and men have benefited greatly from prayer groups that meet at medical centers such as ours. Think of the young man that has let his churchgoing lapse. What about that divorced middle-aged woman searching for answers? Having a pastor to facilitate such a group can show that there is much more to our lives than just those seemingly significant stressors that we incur during our short lives on Earth. Sharing "spiritual moments" can certainly lead to positive life changes, including the following:

- Better sleep
- More peace of mind
- More social interaction
- A safe, supportive environment
- Reduced stress
- Freedom to "breathe"
- A more balanced perspective on life's difficulties
- Trust in something bigger than oneself
- And, of course, improved blood pressure!

After just a few weeks it would certainly not be unusual for prayer group members to begin noticing changes in their medical conditions, particularly if each prayer group member keeps a journal that records progress and thoughts. The stress relief and the easing of anxiety will certainly bring down the participants' blood pressure and ease heart disease symptoms. Imagine the difference in a blood pressure reading of 139/90 versus the much safer 125/80. The group members may still have urges to smoke and overeat, and still experience occasional episodes of anger and stress, but will generally be better able to recognize and change unhealthy emotional and physical habits that contributed to illness. It is my hope that people will feel better, be able to "breathe freely," and manage their blood pressure through faith, prayer, and meditation.

Breathe Deeply: Other Options for Managing Stress

Somewhere you may have come across the concept of deep breathing to relieve stress and promote well-being as well as mental and spiritual growth. The disciplines of yoga and meditation center on correct and conscious breathing. Focusing on your breathing is a way to quiet your mind and allow relaxation as well as meditation.

Not everyone engages in yoga or meditation. However, anyone reading this book that does not have a breathing disorder can benefit from the practice of deep breathing. You can breathe to relax. Making a conscious effort to deepen and slow down your breathing can help you relax. Concentrate on relieving stress by breathing deeply from your stomach, not your chest. When we're upset or stressed, we breathe from the chest. We breathe more rapidly or forget to breathe, period! The denial of oxygen to the blood and the brain is harmful. Also, this type of breathing constricts the blood vessels, which builds blood pressure.

You can reverse this damage and reduce stress by practicing deep breathing when you feel overwhelmed. Visualize your breath as a smooth flow traveling from your nose through your windpipe and lungs and into your abdomen. Expand your abdomen when you inhale. Then, contract your abdomen as you exhale and imagine your breath flowing back smoothly out your nose and mouth. Do this several times and feel the tension ebb away. If you're in the midst of a high-pressure situation that requires you react quickly, do a brief "tension blow-out" with one or two deep breaths. This also works well if you need to eliminate anger in a hurry when your boss or a family member criticizes you and yells at you. In yoga or meditation, you typically breathe in for five or seven counts, hold for five counts, and breathe out for seven counts.

Beyond breathing, here are several other options for managing stress. The goal is to discover what works for you. Be open-minded and willing to experiment. Take action and start enjoying the benefits.

- Simplify your schedule. If you consistently feel rushed, take a few minutes to review your calendar and to-do lists. Look for activities that eat up your time but deliver little value. Schedule less time for such activities, or eliminate them completely.

- Call a friend. People with more social networks usually experience less of the anxiety, depression, and stress that contribute to high blood pressure and heart disease.

- Shift your perspective. When dealing with problems, resist the tendency to complain. Acknowledge your feelings about the situation and then focus on finding solutions.

- If you smoke, quit. Nicotine in cigarettes can actually make you anxious and jittery, although many people say they smoke to relieve stress. Find a healthier means to do so.

- Get a massage, which allows release of stress by stretching and loosening muscles and connective tissues.

- Aim for financial peace. Making money should never be your life goal. Work hard and use your ability and God will provide. Be careful with borrowing money. Don't buy a home if it means getting a mortgage you can't afford—the credit crunch has caused untold woes for millions. Listen to Dave Ramsey for more sound advice.

- A related idea: Do what you love. If you don't love your work, make out a plan so that you can save money, gather your resources, and gain the freedom to do what you are passionate about.

- Stretch and relax. Stand up and stretch each of your muscle groups and focus on releasing the tension in every part of your body.

- Get a pet. Pets have been proven to relieve stress by offering unconditional love as well as physical activity. (Make sure it is the right time, however, as pets may also be the source of tension in a household.)

- Enjoy intimacy with your spouse or partner. As much as we moan and groan about the people we love, having someone to share your worries and joys reduces stress and, in my observation of my friends and family, helps you live longer. In addition, they help you stay true to yourself. My wife reinforces my values, my habits, and my healthy choices.

- Volunteer. This may sound contrary to the advice about not overscheduling, but even something as simple as spending a couple of hours helping out at a charity event can do you a world of good. You'll get a more realistic perspective on your problems, make new friends, and feel a sense of accomplishment. As retired UCLA/Indiana State University basketball coach John Wooden says, "You can't live a perfect day without doing something for someone who will never be able to repay you."

- Give generously to your church and to charity. Even five dollars, some rarely worn clothes from your closet, or a bag of canned goods will help the needy in your community (as well as declutter your home). Doing random acts of kindness actually reduces your stress and makes you feel good. John Wesley, the eighteenth-century founder of the Methodist Church, may have put it best when he said, "Make all you can, save all you can, give all you can!"

- Practice the "it's no big deal" attitude when you're confronted by a rude person, a long line, your child fussing, or the sixteenth time someone interrupts your important presentation.

- Keep a journal of your stresses and also your joys. Pour out all your worries and then describe at least two or three things that made you happy that day, or that you are thankful for. You can even keep a gratitude journal in which you fill a page every day with things you are grateful for—a roof over your head, your family, your eyesight, or whatever you are thankful for.

- Try to do things that make you smile and laugh. This can relieve stress.

- Certainly don't forget to exercise and enjoy. Do something enjoyable, preferably active, whenever possible.

"No" Is Your Friend

In our culture we are constantly pressured to accept things or do things that at another time people would never have dared to ask for.

We are plagued with artificial demands on our time—telemarketing calls, e-mails, media distractions, cell phone calls when we're driving, salespeople who won't leave us alone. Young people today can keep up with a dizzying array of instant-messaging, Facebook, MySpace, text messaging, games and music, as well as online petitions from worthy and not-so-worthy causes. Young people are always "on," interacting with a number of anonymous people they have never even met in person while simultaneously juggling schoolwork, jobs, possible volunteering, and an array of activities. This is why our children are chronically sleep deprived. However, most of them bounce back with the resiliency of youth.

The rest of us can only do so much at one time. We try to keep up a home, pay the bills, raise the kids, and bow to the demands of an increasingly unpredictable and mobile workforce, especially in an economy that seems to change from day to day. We have to go on that sales trip or attend that conference for the third week in a row even though we miss our loved ones and feel guilty about not being there. Psychological stress, as we've seen, leads to unhealthy choices such as alcohol abuse or gambling addiction that can give us (and our loved ones) even more problems, which creates more stress and leads to a vicious cycle. Worry and anxiety become our masters and unleash sickness on us.

Even if we avoid temptation and self-medication, we're vulnerable to the constant sales pitch of our culture: we have to have this home or that stereo, this redecorating job or that car. We need and want to follow this sports team or that TV show. We have to read the books and publications, listen to the music and see the films that all our friends like or that the newspapers and celebrities or other authorities praise. We have to do whatever society is selling us at the time and, simultaneously, try to protect our children from unsafe influences. At times, being "cool" or "in the know" feels like a full-time job.

All of these activities and diversions take us away from what's important in our lives: health, family, friends, work, and spirituality. It's fine to follow sports and attend football games. It's certainly good to volunteer. And it's all right to browse eBay sometimes. It's also all right sometimes to take on extra work to perform well on the job. But beware of falling into a vicious cycle.

Many of us seem to forget the word "no"—even though we may constantly hear it in our lives, we don't think we have the right to use it. I'm here to tell you that "no" can be your friend, and all too often is neglected. You are certainly justified to say "no" to activities that may raise your stress and therefore your blood pressure. These may include helping out at that bake sale when you'd rather not, buying a new car when you want to wait for a better deal, or having lunch with someone who doesn't uplift you.

Saying "no" gives you a feeling of power over your own destiny and well-being. You don't need to shout or put someone down to deliver an effective "no." For most reasonable people, a simple response of "I'd like to, but that's just not possible now" to a request will usually suffice.

All too often when we are confronted with a request or a "hard sell," we find ourselves unprepared and we start to explain rather than assert ourselves. How many times has a salesperson talked you into buying something you didn't exactly want just because the salesperson read indecision in your words and body language as you talked about your budget and your needs?

If you had a blood pressure cuff on your arm during these moments of tension, the monitor reading would likely be increased.

Practice saying no as often as possible so that you can't easily be coerced or talked into something you don't want. If saying "no" isn't an option, here are some strategies to set boundaries, help you avoid stress, and still do what you think you need to do:

- **Negotiate at work.** If you need to refuse taking on more work because you think it's not productive, come up with a list of reasons why the work would cost your employer time and money. Offer to head up a project that will help achieve your boss's goals.

- **Negotiate with family.** If you can't get out of a family or other personal obligation, for example if your mother always nags you to come and visit after work every night, try a compromise. Take your mother out to dinner but tell her you can only stay so long. Set a regular date with your mother once a week. It's harder to say no to family, but when you think you're put-upon, you feel resentment that can only hurt your relationships.

- **Make a trade.** If you have to keep the neighbor's dog for a week and this is the third time you've done it, ask the neighbor to watch your house while you're away on that well-deserved vacation.

- **Counteroffer.** If you can't get out of serving on that committee, offer to do something that you enjoy doing—making five phone calls a week to raise funds, renting an event space, or moderating an online forum.

- **Decide what the activity is worth.** If it's something that will help your goals in the long run, take some deep breaths and agree. Just be sure to balance out your life by exercising for 10 minutes or doing something else you enjoy. Decide what the activity is worth to you.

- **Calculate the cost of living.** If it's a purchase you need to make, decide if the time involved to earn the money and maintain the purchase is worth the benefit of having whatever you're buying.

For more on this concept, I would certainly recommend the book *Boundaries* by Dr. Henry Cloud and Dr. John Townsend. You need to know and respect your limits, including financial ones.

Dollars and Stress

Much has been written about financial freedom and peace of mind. Certainly in today's credit crunch, everyone is even more anxious over money, especially when we spend more than we can afford. Surveys of the American public consistently reveal personal finance and the economy are top sources of stress.

Overspending before the financial collapse worsened some people's current money woes. It was easy to buy a house beyond what a consumer could afford. It was formerly easy to borrow money and to get loans with no income requirements and loans in which both lenders and borrowers knew the lenders couldn't afford the monthly payments. Consumers got adjustable-rate mortgages and bought homes that they couldn't afford to put at least 10 percent down on.

Our parents and grandparents told us that it's easy to get trapped into buying goods you can't pay for today and that will only cost you more in the long run. Consider that the average American has eight credit cards, which means credit card debt! While not all debt is harmful, the fact is that credit card debt usually carries the highest interest rates. We clip coupons to save a quarter, but we sometimes forget to budget for our cell phone and what we can and can't really afford.

Financial expert Suze Orman has a good philosophy: "People first. Then money. Then things." Even professionals with advanced degrees struggle with paying bills; it is easy to overspend on things like eating out and going on vacation.

God has blessed America in many ways, and it is imperative to be financially prudent and exhibit discipline. Think twice about buying a new car instead of depositing a monthly portion of household income into savings and into retirement accounts. That said, you can make all the right decisions and still have occasional worries about money. It's part of life. You, like many people reading this book, played by the rules. You budgeted, saved your money, and still may have been hurt by the financial crisis of recent times.

Unexpected events, such as illness or disability, may put a strain on finances as well as sanity. With health care costs rising, we can protect ourselves by staying as healthy as possible—that means keeping blood pressure in check!

If you do have financial worries, it's important to keep them from poisoning your mind and your health. Your current situation will look even worse if your high blood pressure skyrockets out of control and permanently damages your body. This is the time to put several of the techniques I've suggested into practice. Many of them, such as exercise (at least walking), smiling, laughing, volunteering, and gratitude lists, don't cost anything. You can practice them until you achieve mental peace, which in turn will lower your blood pressure. While you're getting mental clarity, you can make an action plan to save money, invest wisely, and create financial peace even though money may be tight. You know you've weathered similarly tough situations in your past with hard work, optimism, and determination.

You may be angry or resentful about your money problems and about the people who may have caused them. That's normal and human nature. Sometimes you may not even realize the depths of your anger or resentment until you have a meltdown that makes you say words you'll regret. In my experience, turning to faith helps to avoid this.

Time Out!

Even if you don't think you feel resentment, your blood pressure is usually a good barometer of your emotions. Consider the cases you've read about in which a person exhibited no symptoms of heart disease and had none of the traditional risk factors, but experienced a massive coronary attack. In such a heart disease case, cardiologists usually discover through counselors that the heart patient had pent-up emotions from past traumatic events (divorce, death, or loss), old family fights, abuses, hardships, and old slights. Typically the patient comments, "Yes, that happened, and it made me upset, but I got over it."

In these cases, people may think they have moved on, and indeed, they may have made wonderful progress in their lives. However, many psychologists will tell you that moving on outwardly may not be the same thing as emotional acceptance.

There's not enough space in this chapter to provide a thorough psychological discussion—many other people are experts. The purpose of this final chapter is to deal with all the sources of stress that keep your blood pressure high. I've addressed much of what you need to know about bringing down your blood pressure, but this last section will, I hope, help form a total picture of blood pressure treatment in your mind. Many doctors, unfortunately, don't address the role of emotions. Some pioneering literature has opened up the topic, but for the most part, conventional medical wisdom doesn't treat the whole package.

I believe that your medical care should provide personal space, a "time-out," as it were, to address these issues. That's why I'm taking time to enumerate some good emotional habits you can practice to help you recognize and make peace with your feelings. Here are some things that have worked for me and other people I know in the past.

1. When you feel ill or run-down every other week, stop and ask yourself: Is there a physical or an emotional reason I feel this way?

2. If there is no physical cause, examine what you are feeling and thinking. Journaling may help you uncover your real thoughts and cut through the day-to-day mental chatter. One way is to write an unsent letter to someone with whom you are experiencing problems.

3. Monitor what you say to others. By "monitor," I mean observe impartially. Do you notice that you repeatedly talk about unpleasant events in your past? Are you complaining about them without realizing it? An example of this is someone who has been divorced for years but can't let go of past hurts an ex-husband or ex-wife has caused.

4. Identify whether you ever dealt with a specific event emotionally—it doesn't matter if you spent years in therapy. You may not have made peace with whatever sparks your anger, resentment, or even guilt. Guilt can also take a toll on our health.

5. If you feel guilty, ask yourself: Is this appropriate guilt? Were you at fault? If not, can you release that guilt? If so, is there any action you can take to make amends?

6. Write out a list of feelings and events that still cause repressed anger and anxiety. You may need the help of a counselor to help you decide how to approach the people associated with those feelings, especially if those people are part of your life—a husband, wife, parent, sister, brother, boss, or friend.

7. Forgive the hurts. This is easy to say but difficult to do. Many people mistake "forgiving" with "condoning." Forgiving doesn't mean that the hurt (especially in cases of abuse or neglect) was acceptable. It simply means that you let go of your resentment. Forgiveness is a cornerstone of the Christian faith, and Christian counselors can help patients understand the powerful effects of forgiveness on healing.

8. Surround yourself with supportive people who can help you shed your baggage rather than acting as a "misery loves company" society.

9. When your anger and resentment arise, quiet your mind and practice the breathing techniques I discussed earlier. Try to keep your mind clear for at least one minute. If you can take your focus away from your emotions, you can gain a clearer head and perspective before you act destructively toward yourself.

Sometimes, however, all the noise in your mind won't let you be still and calm.

Flow, T'ai Chi, Qigong, and Meditation

I've spoken about how yoga and qigong can help you relax and bring down your blood pressure. I want to address the stress reduction aspects of meditation, t'ai chi, qigong, and yoga.

For instance, qigong is a physical and wellness practice to cleanse and purify the body by accumulating, circulating, and working with qi (or energy) within the body. Qigong can assist you in learning the diaphragmatic breathing I discussed, and as you have seen, proper breathing helps the relaxation response that guards against stress. Qi literally means "breath" in Chinese. Qigong may also help with social connections, since in Chinese culture t'ai chi and qigong are practiced in groups. Social connections help reduce stress, anxiety, and depression. When this reduction is coupled with the natural peace and relaxation promoted by t'ai chi, qigong, and yoga, the de-stressing effect is quite impressive.

T'ai chi and yoga are two of the fastest-growing health and fitness activities in the United States. As I've discussed, t'ai chi also reduces stress through slow, gradual movements. T'ai chi, as an exercise practice, is thought to reduce cortisol and adrenaline, two major stress agents in the body. The effects of t'ai chi aid in clearing the mind and making the body fit so that the individual can engage in meditation. T'ai chi practitioners will tell you that one of the aims of the discipline is to aid in meditation. Since you can't meditate if you're ill or physically uncomfortable, t'ai chi helps you shift into a meditative state, as does yoga. T'ai chi practitioners say that the focus and calmness as well as the stress relief they gain from the meditative aspect of the art help maintain optimum health.

Similarly, even though there are many different styles of yoga, one of the chief aims of yoga is freedom and detachment from worldly distress. I discussed the yoga poses (asanas) that help reduce high blood pressure. Most people in our culture only understand yoga through these poses, but the asanas are purely contemplative in nature, even though performing them seems like quite a physical feat.

However, the awareness you gain from doing the physical yoga helps you become more alert and awake to your own body. Too often we walk around blind to our own physical health until we have pain or we wind up in the ER. Like t'ai chi, part of the goal of yoga is to bring about physical health and mental health so that you can concentrate on meditation. Restorative yoga in particular employs a series of poses with accompanying physical support in order to heal the body from disease and relax the body and mind.

Hatha yoga, the type typically practiced in the West with overemphasis on the physical movements, balances the mind and body through asanas, purification, controlled breathing, and calming the mind through meditation and relaxation. The goal of meditation is to attain mental and spiritual enlightenment. However, many high blood pressure patients will probably not focus on enlightenment as the primary aim when first practicing meditation. Make no mistake: Quieting your mind and letting go of extraneous thoughts is a challenge, especially when so many matters (including your blood pressure reading) compete for your mental attention. At first you won't be able to meditate for more than a minute. This is true of everyone who practices meditation. But with practice, you will improve.

In some hospitals, physicians now offer meditation as an alternative treatment to reduce stress in chronically ill patients, who have depressed immune systems that are particularly vulnerable to stress. Meditation releases the remarkable biochemical and physical changes in the body that make up the relaxation response. Meditation is also supposed to change your brain chemistry and help you adapt better to stressful situations—for example, being in the doctor's office and being anxious about your blood pressure reading.

How does meditation work? Well, of course, these few paragraphs can't possibly cover the wealth of material written on meditation, but here is a simple exercise:

- Sit in a quiet place, preferably early in the morning or late at night. Wear comfortable clothing.
- If you can't sit cross-legged on the floor, sit in a chair or on your bed (if you have limited mobility).
- Start with the breathing techniques I outlined.
- Choose a particular spot in the room and give all your attention to it. Concentrate on nothing but that spot.
- When outside thoughts come, and they will, just let them pass by.
- Sit quietly and silently. Breathe.
- It may be helpful to repeat Scripture or a word such as "peace."
- Do this for one minute and then increase to three or even ten minutes as you progress in your concentration.

I highly recommend meditation, as I do all the stress-relieving techniques and tips in this chapter. You may begin to notice a change in your relaxation response and in your mental and emotional condition once you have practiced medtitation for a while. This is good news for your blood pressure, and that is my goal.

Final De-Stressing Words for Your Optimum Health

If you have resolved to do any or all of the steps in this chapter and this book to bring down your blood pressure, you are to be commended.

You will feel the results of your actions every day of your life. Although you may have some challenges in the beginning, the rewards of increased health, well-being, and quality of life will outmatch the difficulties.

You will experience less overall stress as your mind and body work in harmony, perhaps for the first time in months or years. You'll notice a difference, and not just at the doctor's office.

It's my hope that the resources in the appendices will encourage you to continue to take charge of your health and live the rich, abundant, healthy life you deserve.

Here's to your optimum health!

FAQs ABOUT HIGH BLOOD PRESSURE

General Questions

Q: What is the estimated cost of high blood pressure in the United States?

A: The estimated cost of cardiovascular diseases and stroke in the United States for 2007 is $431.8 billion. This figure includes direct costs (e.g., physicians/other health care providers, hospital/nursing home care, home health care, medications, and medical durables) as well as indirect costs, including lost productivity resulting from morbidity and mortality. Of this figure, at least $66.4 billion, or about 15 percent, can be directly attributed to high blood pressure.

Q: Why is blood pressure one value on one occasion but a different value on another?

A: There may be many answers to this, but one answer may certainly be related to the technique used for checking blood pressure. Although taking a proper blood pressure reading may not be the most difficult thing in the world, a well-trained individual can do so at the optimum level. Often, improper technique leads to inaccurate readings. When you take a wrong reading at home, this may lead you to think incorrectly that blood pressure is within appropriate limits. And of course, you sometimes can experience "white-coat high blood pressure."

On the other hand, when a medical office takes an erroneous reading, this can even have worse implications and lead to incorrect treatment. The proper technique of accurate blood pressure measurement is typically taught very early during medical and nursing training but sometimes gets taken for granted. Although it's okay that some clinics use medical assistants rather than doctors or nurses to take blood pressure, it is important that the measurement is taken by someone well trained!

Q: Is it possible for me to take blood pressure readings at home? You've recommended home blood pressure measuring devices.

A: Fortunately, the technology for accurate and reproducible BP measurement outside the traditional medical environment has improved greatly over the last 30 years. Many convenient, inexpensive, and relatively accurate devices are now available. Even patients with hearing difficulties, problems with hand-eye coordination, and other disabilities can estimate BP with semiautomatic devices that have digital readouts and printers.

Some authorities believe that such devices should be provided to every person with elevated BP, but others are concerned about their use because they have not been commonly used in clinical trials.

Q: What is the proper way to take a blood pressure reading, and when should someone be diagnosed with high blood pressure?

A: To answer the second part of the question, as I mentioned briefly in Chapter 1, high blood pressure is diagnosed only after two readings are elevated on separate occasions. The reason is that blood pressure measurements have much natural variability even with the most accurate device on the market.

Although you can get an accurate blood pressure reading at any given time, blood pressure isn't always the same. It can vary considerably in a short amount of time—sometimes from one heartbeat to the next, depending on body position, breathing rhythm, stress level, physical condition, medications you take, what you eat and drink, and even the time of day.

No matter the technology used for taking blood pressure measurements and no matter the conditions of your body and environment, expert panels have made recommendations regarding how you should measure BP. First and foremost, the blood pressure cuff itself must be appropriately sized for the size of the patient's arm. There are three general sizes to use: one for young children, one for average adults, and a larger cuff for obese adults and others with particularly large arms. Some other controllable factors also lead to incorrect readings. Positioning of the blood pressure cuff as well as proper size are very important. An artery that is key to obtaining accurate blood pressure readings is the brachial artery, and the cuff should be positioned relative to this landmark. The cuff usually indicates which end faces the shoulder and which end faces the elbow. There is usually an arrow on the cuff that points to the brachial artery. Line up this arrow with the brachial artery.

Q: How should I prepare for having my blood pressure checked?
A: Too often, blood pressure readings are made without any concern for prior activity. It's important to avoid caffeine, alcohol, and tobacco for at least 30 minutes before a blood pressure measurement. The stimulants caffeine and tobacco in particular may acutely increase blood pressure.

You may think you're safer drinking several glasses of water or juice before a blood pressure reading. However, having a full bladder and needing a bowel movement may also affect blood pressure control. Make sure, however, that you are properly hydrated.

Heat also affects your readings. This is one reason that signs posted above public hot tubs warn about prolonged soaking. High surrounding temperature typically causes blood pressure to drop as blood vessels dilate in order to keep body temperature constant. That drop in blood pressure can cause you to faint, especially if you are already taking anti-high-blood-pressure medication.

A properly recorded blood pressure should only be taken after at least five minutes of comfortable rest. You may find it helpful to relax and take several deep breaths. A mini meditation may also calm your body and dilate your blood vessels. Then, as I mentioned in Chapter 1, have your blood pressure taken (or take it at home) at the level of the heart and the arm. Taking the blood pressure below that level may lead to falsely high readings, and the opposite is true of taking the blood pressure with the arm positioned above the heart and the other arm. Tip: Measure BP in both arms at first and in the arm with the higher BP thereafter if the difference is greater than 10/5 mmHg.

Q: What does hydration have to do with blood pressure?
A: Blood pressure is usually lowest at night and rises sharply on waking. With poor hydration, the levels fall drastically. You need to drink plenty of fluids before you have your blood pressure checked or you take it yourself.

Preventing dehydration is easy if you follow fluid intake guidelines from the Institute of Medicine for "healthy sedentary adults living in temperate climates" (i.e., with season changes). Men should take in approximately 125 ounces or 3.7 liters of water per day from all dietary sources. Most women, on the other hand, should get about 91 ounces (or 2.7 liters) of water per day from all dietary sources. Food intake actually usually supplies about 20 percent of our daily fluid intake, so that means men need to drink approximately three quarts per day and women over two quarts per day. Low-sugar fruit ices, sugar-free frozen pops, and sugar-free gelatin desserts are good supplements to increase amount of overall fluid intake.

Q: How do home blood pressure readings compare?
A: Several reports show a benefit to supplementing clinical blood pressure readings with home self-monitoring. Home readings can be helpful in evaluating symptoms, especially ones that aren't chronic, that are suggestive of high blood pressure. Often these symptoms aren't present during the few minutes of a typical physician's-office visit. In fact, when done correctly, home monitoring can actually save quite a bit in costs related to follow-up office visits.

Because people typically feel less stressed taking BP at home, BP readings are typically lower than measurements taken in the traditional medical environment, even in persons with normal blood pressure. Also, routine home BP monitoring gives you an advantage when you undertake a blood pressure–lowering plan. This is primarily because you are paying close attention to the condition. I concur with many physicians who say an individual prognosis is better predicted by home readings than by one or two "casual" office BP measurements.

Long-term study has shown that people with much lower home BP readings suffer fewer major cardiovascular events than do people who have elevated readings both in the office and at home. Thus, if the home BP reading differs widely from the office BP reading, this is possibly a favorable sign of improved hearth health.

In addition, home blood pressure monitoring is a practical way to evaluate therapies for lowering blood pressure and to assess BP response out of the office prior to using ambulatory blood pressure monitoring. Blood pressure checks at home may also be especially helpful for smokers and patients who don't always comply with physician instructions.

I will advise that home readings should be interpreted cautiously, carefully, and conservatively. Many of the factors that contribute to blood pressure variability are more difficult to control in the home environment—such as food and alcohol ingestion, activity levels, and stress. If home readings are taken, the home measuring device should be calibrated against the standard clinical BP measuring device in a physician's office. Any device that is used at home should pass the Aggressive Standards for Advancement of Medical Instruments. Home measurements, however, should *never* be a *substitute* for recommended checks in a medical setting.

Q: What should I look for when monitoring blood pressure at home?
A: If you record home measurements of greater than 135/85 mmHg, you have high blood pressure. However, false readings can occur. You should use the same techniques at home that are used in the doctor's office, most importantly sitting quietly for two to five minutes first and making sure that the cuff covers 80 percent of the circumference of the arm. Also, you may find it beneficial to keep a record of the blood pressures measured and the time and date they are taken to share with the doctor at the next appointment.

Q: What is "ambulatory blood pressure monitoring"?
A: Since we don't sit still with BP monitors attached to our arms all day, scientists have devised another way to measure blood pressure. This method uses automated blood pressure measurement over a 24-hour period during a person's usual daily activities. Scientists think of ambulatory blood pressure monitoring (ABPM) devices as "the gold standard," the best method of measuring blood pressure in controlled research trials. ABMP devices are beginning to have a greater place in clinical practice in the United States because insurers have increased their reimbursement for ABPM technology.

The advantages of ABPM devices include the number of measurements obtained during a 24-hour period, including during sleep and daily activities. ABPM can identify and diagnose white-coat high blood pressure. However, a few of the disadvantages include the cost, limited availability, inconsistent conditions, disruption of daily life because of noise or discomfort, and lack of defined "normal values." Also, there are no standard guidelines for treatment or long-term studies demonstrating the superiority of this practice.

Q: I have been diagnosed with high blood pressure and am following the recommendations I was given. When and how often should I go back for a checkup?

A: A few recommendations can be made on follow-ups based on initial blood pressure measurements for adults. Even if the initial blood pressure measurement (measured in mmHg) is normal, it is recommended that you have it checked again in one year. If the initial blood pressure measurement is pre–high blood pressure (please see Chapter 1 for this definition), a follow-up should be made sooner. Here are some other frequent scenarios, although it is important to follow your doctor's specific instructions:

- If the initial blood pressure is Stage 1, a confirmation follow-up should be done within two months.
- If the initial blood pressure reading reveals Stage 2 high blood pressure, an evaluation or referral to a source of care should take place within a month.
- If the blood pressure is greater than 180/110 mmHg, evaluation and treatment should take place within a week if not immediately.

It is important for physicians and other clinicians to monitor and anticipate problems complying with prescribed treatment, especially for young men. Anyone who has high blood pressure and/or is being evaluated for high blood pressure should always bring all medicines from all physicians and other sources (prescription, complementary, or over-the-counter) to each visit for review. This helps a physician to determine if blood pressure is being affected by unnecessary causes. Fortunately, many patients with high blood pressure are treated in primary care with well-controlled blood pressure. However, with surveys estimating that only about 30 percent of all Americans who have high blood pressure are controlling the condition, physicians need to strive in their practices to ensure that all patients with high blood pressure have it under control.

Q: Can my blood pressure be too low?
A: At the other end of the spectrum, we have mentioned low blood pressure briefly. Some people who are healthy, eat a balanced diet, and exercise regularly but still have blood pressure regularly on the low side wonder if they should be concerned. On the contrary, they should ask for a reduced rate on their life insurance. If you feel healthy, having a relatively low blood pressure is good for the cardiovascular sys-

tem, since it puts less stress on the blood vessels. However, low blood pressure can indicate a few disorders in people that are not healthy.

You can never be too rich, too thin, or too-low-blood-pressure . . . right? Well, not exactly. That's where this business of measuring blood pressure gets tricky (as if it wasn't already). Low blood pressure, called hypotension, is much harder to quantify, but it is worth a mention. Some experts define low blood pressure as readings lower than 90 systolic or 60 diastolic. Unlike your numbers for high blood pressure, you only need to have one number in the low range for your blood pressure to be considered lower than normal. If your systolic pressure is a perfect 115 but your diastolic pressure is 50, the medical establishment judges that you have lower than normal pressure.

Yet as with much medical data, these numbers can be misleading simply because one size does not fit all. What's considered low blood pressure for you may be normal for someone else. For that reason, doctors often consider chronically low blood pressure too low only if it causes noticeable symptoms.

On the other hand, a sudden fall in blood pressure can be dangerous. A change of just 20 mmHg, for example, a drop from 130 systolic to 110 systolic (top number) can cause dizziness and fainting when the brain fails to receive an adequate supply of blood. And big plunges, especially those caused by uncontrolled bleeding, severe infections, or allergic reactions can be life-threatening.

Q: What causes low blood pressure?
A: Athletes as well as people who exercise regularly tend to have lower blood pressure than do people who aren't as fit. So, in general, do nonsmokers and people who eat well and maintain a normal weight. However, in some instances, low blood pressure can be a sign of serious, even life-threatening disorders. Authorities such as the American Heart Association advise possible causes of low blood pressure, such as the following:

1. The first and second trimesters of pregnancy
2. Medications such as those used to treat Parkinson's disease, Viagra (particularly in combination with nitroglycerine), and even heart medication such as beta-blockers
3. Narcotic and alcohol abuse
4. Heart problems

5. Endocrine problems
6. Dehydration
7. Blood loss
8. Septic shock (blood infection) and anaphylaxis (as in peanut or food allergies)
9. Nutritional deficiencies
10. Postprandial low blood pressure found in adults with high blood pressure or automatic nervous system disorders (such as Parkinson's disease)
11. Postural low blood pressure, which occurs in adults who stand abruptly from a sitting or prone position and can be caused by conditions including heatstroke, dehydration, heart problems, and excessive bed rest as well as certain medications such as ACE inhibitors and medication for Parkinson's disease
12. Neurally mediated low blood pressure occurring in young people who stand for long periods

Interestingly, high blood pressure is connected to low blood pressure in at least one of the causes, so let's return to our "King Kong" of diseases.

Q: My doctor referred me to a high blood pressure specialist at a high blood pressure clinic. Is this a good move?
A: Sometimes it may be necessary for your doctor to refer you to a high blood pressure specialist. This is not because he or she doesn't want to deal with the issue. It simply means that the provider is trying to get you to the most knowledgeable person to help your condition.

A local high blood pressure clinic may be an obvious place for a doctor to refer a patient, but not all general practitioners have such a local clinic. Where there is no specialist clinic, your doctor will most likely refer you to the local cardiologist. But your local cardiologist may not have any specialist training or an interest in high blood pressure, and may actually have little relative experience managing high blood pressure. In that case, a better alternative may be a local vascular or stroke physician, an elderly care physician, or a general practitioner with a specific interest (GPSI). Many GPSIs have completed training in high blood pressure treatment.

The specialist, GPSI, or other doctor needs to have as many facts on hand as possible when they see the patient. If they have to arrange tests, this just delays implementing treatment. A local specialist or GPSI will often want or need to see the results of the following:

- A prevention screen, including lipids and blood glucose.
- Routine lab tests such as microalbuminuria.
- 24-hour urine test (for electrolytes, kidney function, etc.).
- Routine electrocardiogram (ECG), especially when left ventricular hypertrophy has been previously seen, with a copy of the new ECG to be sent with the referral.

Q: I don't have high blood pressure right now. Is there any reason for me to pay attention to it?
A: You're reading this book, so the odds are that you are concerned or somewhat curious, with good reason. Primary prevention of high blood pressure can improve quality of life and costs associated with medical management of high blood pressure and its complications. A viable strategy for the general population would be to reduce blood pressure in those with higher-than-optimal levels but below the cut points for diagnosis.

Recent research shows that higher-than-normal blood pressures that didn't meet the criteria for high blood pressure were associated with an increased risk of cardiovascular disease. A downward shift of 3 mmHg in systolic (top number) BP would decrease the mortality from stroke by 8 percent and from coronary heart disease by 5 percent. People at highest risk should be strongly encouraged to adopt healthier lifestyle changes, which are essential for both prevention and management of high blood pressure.

Q: What is secondary high blood pressure and why should I be worried?
A: Other conditions can cause high blood pressure. As you read in Chapter 1, this book focuses on primary high blood pressure. Secondary high blood pressure, however, is of particular importance and needs to be explained.

When something goes wrong in one part of your body, a ripple effect can create problems elsewhere, such as high blood pressure. In fact, 5 to 10 percent of high blood pressure cases are caused by an underlying condition, according to the American Heart Association. This type of high blood pressure, known as secondary hypertension, tends to appear suddenly.

Various conditions can cause secondary high blood pressure. However, there's good news: Treating these underlying conditions can control, or cure, your high blood pressure. This reduces the risk of serious complications that include heart disease, kidney failure, and stroke.

Q: What are the possible causes of secondary high blood pressure?
A: Here is a partial list, many of which involve the kidney(s):

- **Diabetic nephropathy:** Your kidneys contain millions of tiny blood vessels that filter waste from your blood and eliminate it in your urine. But diabetes can damage this delicate filtering system. In fact, diabetic nephropathy is the most common type of kidney failure, which is nearly always associated with high blood pressure. The high blood pressure can be treated with diet, exercise, and medication. If your kidney function dips too low, you may need dialysis or a kidney transplant.
- **Polycystic kidney disease:** In this inherited condition, cysts in the kidneys disrupt normal function and raise blood pressure. The high blood pressure can be treated with diet, exercise, and medication. The polycystic disease may ultimately require dialysis or a kidney transplant.
- **Glomerular disease:** Your kidneys filter waste and sodium using microscopic filters called glomeruli. Inflammation of these filters is called glomerulonephritis. If the inflamed glomeruli can't function normally, you may develop high blood pressure. The high blood pressure can be treated with diet, exercise, and medication. Glomerulonephritis may be treated with medication, dialysis, or a kidney transplant.
- **Hydronephrosis:** When certain parts of one or both kidneys become plugged, it causes urine flow blockage, which raises blood pressure. Some blockages resolve without treatment, but others require drainage or surgery. Once the blockage is removed, blood pressure often returns to normal.
- **Renovascular high blood pressure:** This is a type of secondary high blood pressure caused by narrowing (stenosis) of one or both renal arteries. Renovascular high blood pressure can cause severe hypertension and irreversible kidney damage. It's often caused by the same type of fatty plaques that can damage your coronary arteries (atherosclerosis) or a condition in which the

muscle and fibrous tissues of the renal artery wall thicken and harden into rings (fibromuscular dysplasia). In mild cases, the high blood pressure may be treated with diet, exercise, and medication while kidney function is simply monitored. In more severe cases, the doctor may open clogged arteries with a procedure known as angioplasty. Wire mesh tubes (stents) may be used to hold the arteries open. Another option is to surgically bypass blood flow around the affected arteries. Once blood flow to the kidneys improves, blood pressure usually returns to normal.

- **Cushing's syndrome:** Corticosteroid medications, a pituitary tumor, or other factors cause the adrenal glands to produce too much of the hormone cortisol. This raises blood pressure. Treatment may include surgery, radiation therapy, or medication to return both cortisol and blood pressure to normal.
- **Aldosteronism:** A tumor in the adrenal gland, increased growth of normal cells, or other factors cause the adrenal glands to release an excessive amount of the hormone aldosterone. This makes your kidneys retain salt and water and lose too much potassium, which, as you have read, raises blood pressure. Treatment may include medication to block the action of aldosterone and surgery to remove a tumor in the adrenal gland, complemented by a proper diet, exercise, and medication to treat the high blood pressure.
- **Pheochromocytoma:** This rare tumor in the adrenal gland increases production of the hormones adrenaline and noradrenaline, which can lead to persistent high blood pressure or marked fluctuations in blood pressure. Surgery to remove the tumor returns blood pressure to normal.
- **Hypothyroidism:** The thyroid gland doesn't produce enough thyroid hormone, which can cause high blood pressure. Hypothyroidism may have various causes, including inflammation, surgery, radiation treatment, certain medications, or pituitary problems. Treatment with synthetic thyroid hormones usually returns blood pressure to normal.
- **Hyperthyroidism:** The thyroid gland produces too much thyroid hormone, which increases the activity of epinephrine and norepinephrine, which in turn can increase blood pressure. Treatment may include medication, radioactive iodine therapy, or surgery, all of which can restore normal blood pressure.

- **Hyperparathyroidism:** The parathyroid glands regulate levels of calcium and phosphorus in your body. If the glands secrete too much parathyroid hormone, the amount of calcium in your blood rises, which triggers a rise in blood pressure. Treatment is typically removal of the parathyroid glands, which often returns blood pressure to normal.

- **Coarctation of the aorta:** With this congenital defect of the body's main artery (aorta), a constriction (coarctation) in part of the aorta forces the heart to pump harder to get blood through the aorta and to the rest of your body. This, in turn, raises blood pressure, particularly in your arms. Surgery to repair the aorta can restore normal blood pressure.

- **Sleep apnea:** Your breathing repeatedly stops and starts during sleep. The repeated episodes of oxygen deprivation may damage the cellular lining of the blood vessel walls, which may deprive blood vessels of the elasticity they need to regulate blood pressure. Treating sleep apnea with a pressure mask, nasal devices, surgery, weight loss, or other steps can help control the high blood pressure.

- **Obesity:** As you gain weight, the amount of blood circulating through your body increases. This puts added pressure on your artery walls. In addition, excess weight often is associated with an increase in heart rate and a reduction in the capacity of your blood vessels to transport blood. All of these factors can increase blood pressure.

- **Medications, supplements, and illicit drugs:** Various prescription medications from pain relievers to antidepressants and drugs used after organ transplants can cause or aggravate high blood pressure. Birth control pills, decongestants, and certain herbal supplements, including ginseng and St. John's wort, may have the same effect. Many illicit drugs, such as cocaine and methamphetamine, also increase blood pressure.

High Blood Pressure in Men versus Women

Q: Is it true that hot flashes increase blood pressure?
A: New research indicates hot flashes are, in fact, associated with an increase in blood pressure and a decrease in memory as well as quality of sleep.

Among the recent studies linking health problems to hot flashes is one from Weill Medical College of Cornell University, which showed that hot flashes are associated with an increase in blood pressure. The all-female survey revealed that participants who had experienced hot flashes in the two previous weeks had significantly higher systolic blood pressure (the top number) than those who had not.

Thus, your doctor needs to follow your menopausal symptoms and therapy closely as part of your blood pressure treatment. You can reduce or eliminate the effects of hot flashes with the following steps:

- Stop smoking. Tobacco is associated with increased hot flashes.
- Eat more legumes and vegetables.
- Eat one to two teaspoons of ground flaxseed daily.
- Eat more soy foods, especially those that contain naturally occurring phytoestrogens. Tempeh, tofu, soy milk, and soy nuts as well as edamame are good sources.
- Exercise!
- Practice the de-stressing techniques in Chapter 8.
- Keep your bedroom cool at night.
- Wear loose clothing and dress in layers so you can remove one if necessary.
- Use alternative therapies only under a doctor's supervision.
- If necessary, avoid alcohol, spicy foods, hot drinks, and caffeine, which trigger hot flashes in some women.

Q: How does high blood pressure affect men?

A: We mentioned men's sexual function in Martin's story in Chapter 1. Experts don't know exactly how high blood pressure causes erectile dysfunction and impotence. One leading theory is that the excess pressure in the blood vessels actually causes damage to small arteries in the penis, according to Dr. Craig Weber. Normally, these arteries dilate in response to sexual stimulation, allowing more blood to flow into the spongy tissue of the penis to produce an erection.

Experts think that excessive pressure on these arteries may cause tiny rips, which the body then repairs. In response to these rips, the healed arteries become thicker, allowing them to better resist further damage. These thicker arteries, though, aren't able to respond as fast, or as completely, to demands for extra blood, so they become a sort of dam in the flow of blood to the erectile tissues of the penis.

One problem with this theory is that some studies seem to show that how long a patient has had high blood pressure is not as important for predicting the risk of erectile dysfunction as is the actual severity of the high blood pressure. In other words, someone who has had moderate high blood pressure (140/90) for 20 years sometimes appears to be at lower risk for erectile dysfunction than a young man who has had very serious high blood pressure (160/100) for only a few months. In light of this, other theories of how high blood pressure contributes to erectile dysfunction have been proposed.

Regardless of the cause, the interruption in your sex life, and the loss of health benefits and intimacy, is certainly serious enough to take care of your ticker and get regular blood pressure checkups.

Q: Are women better at managing high blood pressure than men?
A: Ironically, men have in the past been more likely to take care of themselves than women in this regard. Women underestimate their risk for high blood pressure and heart disease, and often put their health secondary to family, job, career, volunteering, and all their other obligations. Let's put our women first! The NHLBI Heart Truth campaign aims to reach women between the ages of 40 and 60 and women of color who have the highest risk factors for heart disease. The American Heart Association has designated February Red Dress Month, which focuses on heart disease as the leading cause of death in women. Because of such initiatives, women are now more aware of their risk.

Spousal support (and relatives' and friends' support) can make all the difference in helping men and women exercise, manage stress, cut down on salt, and maintain a healthy diet.

Health Habits

Q: What does oral hygiene have to do with high blood pressure and heart disease?
A: You've repeatedly heard it from your dentist since your very first teeth cleaning and checkup: Brush twice a day and don't forget to floss. But this advice may contribute even more to your health and savings than just a mouth full of cavity-free teeth.

Research demonstrates a connection between gum disease and cardiovascular disease. This information is relatively recent and less well established when compared with other known risk factors for heart disease such as high blood pressure and high cholesterol, but it is solid.

Gum or periodontal disease is a collection of inflammatory diseases affecting the tissues that surround and support the teeth. The bone reduction related to periodontal disease may lead to loosening and, if periodontal disease is untreated, eventual loss of teeth. Bacteria that adhere to and grow on tooth surfaces, especially in areas under the gum line, cause periodontal disease.

These bacteria can gain access to the bloodstream, triggering inflammation in the body. As with any infectious disease, your body reacts. An inflammatory reaction can be severe with infections such as the flu, in which a fever and increased white blood cell count help fight the illness. With periodontal disease, the level of inflammation is much less severe and is usually not high enough to cause these systemic symptoms. However, the chronic low level of inflammation may be enough to bother the blood vessels and help trigger vascular disease. White blood cells present in atherosclerotic, or hardened, blood vessels sense the low-level reaction and produce a variety of factors that may worsen the disease process.

Also, some evidence suggests that periodontal bacteria can attach to the fatty plaques in blood vessels, amplifying the inflammatory process, which can lead to heart attack or stroke. This mechanism is similar to periodontal bacteria attaching to heart valves, which can lead to a serious infection of the heart lining known as endocarditis.

We've mentioned C-reactive protein (CRP). Patients with periodontal disease typically have elevated CRP levels, an independent risk predictor of cardiovascular disease. CRP can be detected via a blood test that detects the level of inflammation in the body.

Q: You talked about the importance of maintaining a healthy weight for optimum blood pressure. How do I know if I am overweight and/ or obese—by looking in the mirror?
A: Using a mirror may offer an idea, but too often people are either overly critical or they deny any problem.

As we saw in Chapter 2, body mass index (BMI) helps determine if someone is overweight. Doctors use BMI and waist circumference measurement to rule whether someone is overweight and/or obese.

One way to determine if you may need to shed a few "lbs" for your health is to simply check your belt—literally. This may sound rude, or even a bit simple, but the truth is that one of the best indicators we have is waist size. Now, there is a certain place to measure, so wearing your belt around your hips doesn't count. In general, take the measurement around the largest part of your belly across the belly button for a fairly good estimate. Men should have a waist no more than 40 inches and women should not exceed a waist of 35 inches. Although this does not mean that being an inch or two below these cutoffs is necessarily optimal, above these sizes, you significantly increase your chance for type 2 diabetes and ultimately heart disease. Waist size is very closely related to what is called "insulin resistance," which seems to be a risk factor for high blood pressure and also heart disease.

Another easy way to determine if you need to lose weight is to calculate your BMI to see if your weight falls into the healthy, overweight, or obese range. Use this simple formula to calculate your BMI: (weight in pounds $\times$ 703) $\div$ (height in inches squared). To calculate the square of a number, multiply it by itself. In an example BMI calculation, for someone 5 feet, 7 inches tall, weighing 150 lbs, the equation looks like this: $(150 \times 703) \div (67 \times 67) = 105,450 \div 4,489 = 23.5$.

If you are overweight or obese, a weight loss of about 22 pounds (10 kg) can result in a systolic blood pressure drop of up to 10 mmHg or more, depending on the level of a patient's obesity. Most people can lose that amount of weight relatively easily.

Q: How does a vegetarian diet help lower blood pressure?
A: Factors other than dietary fat, such as increased potassium levels (see Chapter 3), appear to lower blood pressure in vegans. Although dietary lipids do not seem to directly affect blood pressure, they strongly affect CVD risk. Thus, a completely vegetarian diet with an adequate complement of protein is recommended for preventing complications from hypertension and CVD. An olive oil–enriched diet has been shown to decrease blood pressure drug usage drastically, and as we've seen, soy protein is another factor that may contribute to the lowering of blood pressure. Soy isoflavones may also be beneficial for menopausal women.

Q: How much alcohol does it take to raise blood pressure?
A: My fellow physicians have reported that 5 to 7 percent of the high blood pressure in the population is due to alcohol consumption. This

may depend on the individual. However, as a rule, in men an intake of more than two drinks per day (a total of more than three ounces of alcohol) is the amount that raises blood pressure. Therefore, to prevent high blood pressure, men should consume no more than two drinks per day. In women and lighter-weight persons, no more than one drink a day is recommended.

What counts as a drink? Let's test your alcohol IQ as it pertains to blood pressure. Think in your mind . . . is the answer true or false?

1. People with high blood pressure don't have to limit the amount of alcoholic beverages they drink.
2. Alcoholic drinks contain calories, which is another good reason to cut back on them if you're trying to lose weight and control high blood pressure.
3. A 12-ounce can of beer counts as one drink, the same as 5 ounces of wine or 1½ ounces of whiskey.

I hope you answered False, True, and True respectively. If so, you have a high IQ as it relates to blood pressure and risk factors.

Q: Are headaches related to blood pressure?

A: Headaches can be devastating, but they can also just be a nuisance that inhibits our best function. Headaches have also been associated with high blood pressure. The link between headaches, including migraine headaches, and high blood pressure is controversial. Research seems to agree that migraines are linked to a consistent systolic (top number) reading of 140 or a diagnosis of severe high blood pressure. Mild high blood pressure doesn't produce headaches.

If you have migraines and severe high blood pressure, proper eating habits, such as those described in this book, can help maintain good flow of energy and blood to the head. Also, eating frequent smaller meals to feed the brain more often certainly makes sense—selecting natural foods with no additives is recommended, of course. A migraine prevention diet is similar to a heart disease prevention diet.

To avoid migraines, eat fiber-rich foods. In addition, green leafy vegetables, parsley, green tea, onions, ginger, pearl barley, carrots, prunes, buckwheat, peach kernels, and almonds have all been recommended by nutrition experts for headache relief, as well as chrysanthemum flowers (these are not just for decoration).

On the other side of the coin, headache sufferers may want to avoid certain food triggers that include alcohol, chocolate, MSG, nitrates, sulfites, sugar, salt, spicy foods, heavy starchy foods, caffeine, and fried/greasy foods—many of the same things that can raise high blood pressure. This does not mean people who have migraines and severe high blood pressure need to avoid everything on this list. These are simply food triggers to watch for.

As with high blood pressure, headaches decrease in intensity with motion. Stretching and (if possible) taking a light walk in fresh air can nip a headache in the bud. This will stimulate blood flow and allow more oxygen to the head. The relaxation techniques discussed in Chapter 8 (t'ai chi and meditation) are also therapeutic.

It is important to visit your physician an emergency room immediately should you ever experience severe, debilitating headaches that don't respond to simple over-the-counter medication—or wake up in the middle of the night with an excruciating headache.

Q: How is fatigue related to blood pressure?
A: Fatigue commonly occurs with high blood pressure. On the other hand, blood pressure that is too low may also cause fatigue, lightheadedness, and depression.

As with headaches, fatigue that interferes with your daily routine can be conquered using the same methods as those used to treat high blood pressure. There are certainly numerous options to help regain the physical and mental energy needed to enjoy life to its fullest, no matter your sex or age. For example, learn to eat foods that increase your energy levels. An emphasis on consumption of vegetables, whole grains, and healthy oils is the foundation of this approach. You see, different kinds of foods are converted to energy at different speeds. For example, simple sugar forms (e.g., candy) can provide a quick lift, followed by a low. On the other hand, however, unprocessed foods (such as whole grains and healthy unsaturated fats) will provide sustained energy throughout the day. Eat small, frequent meals throughout the day to provide a steady supply of fuel that reduces your brain's perception of fatigue. Adding a daily multivitamin will ensure that you get the vitamins and minerals you need.

Don't let yourself get caught up in buying those energy supplements at the grocery or gas station checkout. Most of these supplements merely contain a form of caffeine like coffee, and use of these quick fixes can often lead to worsening fatigue problems when any positive effects wear off. In addition, as you learned in Chapter 7, certain stimulants can actually add stress to the heart and your circulatory (blood) system.

As mentioned earlier, stress often contributes to fatigue. Accordingly, relaxation therapy (e.g., self-hypnosis, yoga, massage, aromatherapy, and t'ai chi) can be an effective tool for reducing stress and naturally boosting your energy. Also, Harvard experts recommend the "progressive muscle relaxation" technique. This involves systematically tightening and releasing sets of muscles, beginning with your toes and progressing up your legs, torso, hands, and arms. I would recommend Harvard Health Publications' *Boosting Your Energy* report to help you take the first steps toward an energized life.

Q: What is an aortic aneurysm? Should I get screened?
A: It is a bulge in a section of the aorta, the largest artery in the body. High blood pressure and atherosclerosis (hardening of the arteries) weaken the artery walls. When this is combined with the wear and tear that naturally occurs with aging, an aneurysm can occur. Because this area of the artery becomes weak, it can rupture. A ruptured aneurysm causes severe pain and bleeding. It often leads to death within minutes to hours.

Most aortic aneurysms don't cause symptoms. People who do have symptoms complain of belly, chest, or back pain and discomfort. Aneurysms are often found and diagnosed by chance during exams or tests done for other reasons. However, they may be found during a screening test. Routine screening tests for aneurysms are recommended for men who are:

- Ages 65 to 75 and have ever smoked.
- At least 60 years old and have a first-degree relative who has had an aneurysm.

If you do not fall into these categories, however, ask your doctor what is right for you.

Appendix A

NUTRITIONAL BENEFITS OF SUPERFOODS

"SUPERFOOD" HAS BECOME a buzzword in health today, and like so many popularized phrases, has lost its meaning to advertising. So-called superfood products line grocery store and health food store shelves. Some are more effective than others. Although I won't devote much space here to discussing açai berries, mangosteen, dragonfruit and other exotic foods that are popular, I will make mention of one you may not have heard of—cupuaçu. It is a powerful and delicious berry, and although further research is needed, cupuaçu appears to have great potential to impact health. It can be found in AS-10, a product available on my Web site at http://www.shop.youroptimumhealth.net.

Our goal has been to take a back-to-basics approach to bringing down high blood pressure. Here are some staple superfoods to keep around—most are fairly simple but important for good health.

- **Egg Whites**

In addition to supplying needed protein, egg whites contain much-needed vitamins. They are a powerhouse of nutrients that can keep your blood pressure low and keep your weight down because they satisfy your hunger. In particular, egg whites are rich in vitamin D and zinc, which lower blood pressure.

- **Apples**

The saying "an apple a day" has a lot of truth.

Apples may reduce the risk of certain cancers such as colorectal, largely because of fiber content, which helps regulate bowel movements.

Certain compounds found in apples may be cancer-protective and demonstrate antioxidant activity.

Apples may also help with heart disease, weight loss, and controlling cholesterol. Apples do not have any cholesterol, and they do have fiber, which reduces cholesterol by preventing reabsorption. Whether you choose the Red Delicious, Macintosh, or Granny Smith variety, you'll find apples are bulky for their caloric content like most fruits and vegetables.

You can snack on apples anywhere, anytime.

- **Dried Fruits**

Dried fruits' water content shrinks in comparison to fresh fruit. This makes the nutrients in dried fruit more concentrated. Dried fruits are rich in vitamin A and several B vitamins, and are a good supply of minerals such as iron and potassium. Because dried fruits are high in natural sugars, opt for dried fruit products that don't contain added sugars.

- **Dark Green Leafy Vegetables**

Spinach, kale, romaine lettuce, leaf lettuce, mustard greens, collard greens, chicory, and Swiss chard are excellent sources of **fiber, folate,** and a wide range of **carotenoids** such as lutein and zeaxanthin, along with saponins and flavonoids.

It has been reported that foods containing carotenoids may protect against certain types of cancer. Saponins are thought to fight cholesterol and prevent inflammation that can lead to heart disease.

- **Nuts: Peanuts, Walnuts, Pecans, Almonds, and Nut Butters**

Nuts contain plant sterols and are one of the best plant sources of protein. Nuts contain magnesium, antioxidants such as vitamin E and selenium, folic acid (peanuts), and zinc. Nuts are high in monounsaturated fats and polyunsaturated omega-3 fatty acids that help lower cholesterol and reduce the risk of heart disease. In addition, nuts provide an excellent dose of protein and are rich in fiber.

Nut butters such as almond, cashew, hazelnut, and pistachio are rich in unsaturated fats. Almond butter is a good source of magnesium.

- **Soy**

Soybeans are high in magnesium. There is much debate over which forms of soy protein are best. Some authorities tell you to avoid the commercially produced American soy milk products, soy meal bars, soy nuts, soy cheese, and so on, and most soy sauces are high in sodium. However, edamame, tofu, some soy milks (enriched with essential vitamins), and several forms of soy protein can help maintain your normal blood pressure.

- **Quinoa**

This South American grain contains a balanced set of all nine essential amino acids, which makes it an unusually complete protein source. In fact, one cup of cooked quinoa equals eight grams of protein, higher than in most other grains. It is a good source of dietary fiber and phosphorus and is high in magnesium and iron. Quinoa is easy to digest. In addition, it's gluten-free, which is beneficial to people with sensitivities.

- **Flaxseeds**

Flaxseeds contain high levels of lignans and omega-3 fatty acids. In addition to the heart health benefits of omega-3 fatty acids, lignans may benefit the heart. Lignans also possess anticancer properties. Studies performed on mice found reduced growth in specific types of tumors. In addition, initial studies suggest that flaxseed taken in the diet may benefit individuals with certain types of breast and prostate cancers.

Flaxseed has other health benefits. It may lessen the severity of diabetes by stabilizing blood-sugar levels. There is some support for the use of flaxseed as a laxative due to its dietary fiber content.

As a caution, excessive consumption without liquid can result in intestinal blockage. Consuming large amounts of flaxseed can impair the effectiveness of certain oral medications, due to its fiber content.

- **Natural Oatmeal**

Daily consumption of a bowl of oatmeal can lower blood cholesterol, due to its soluble fiber content. The popularity of oatmeal and other oat products increased after the January 1997 decision by the Food and Drug Administration that food with oat bran or rolled oats can carry a label claiming it may reduce the risk of heart disease when combined with a low-fat diet. This is because of the beta-glucan in the oats.

Rolled oats have also long been a staple of many athletes' diets, especially weight trainers, given oatmeal's high content of complex carbohydrates and water-soluble fiber that encourages slow digestion and stabilizes blood-glucose levels.

Oatmeal contains more B vitamins and calories than other kinds of cereals. Cooked oatmeal has a lower glycemic index value than has uncooked, because cooking releases water-soluble fiber from the grain.

- **Fat-Free Cottage Cheese**

As advertised, this superfood is obviously low in fat, and is also low in carbohydrates while high in protein. Fat-free cottage cheese is rich in calcium. One serving generally has about 80 calories. You can buy low sodium varieties, which are of course best for blood pressure.

- **Cupuaçu**

The cupuaçu tree is common throughout the Amazon basin and Brazil's northeastern regions. Cupuaçu belongs to the same genus as cocoa, the raw ingredient of chocolate, and therefore shares many of the same properties such as its rich taste and high flavonoid content. Claims that the fruit improves circulation, lowers blood pressure, and stimulates mental function are all promising, although more research is needed. Cupuaçu is a natural source of phosphorus, fiber, the B vitamins, and vitamins A and C. Cupuaçu contains unique antioxidant phytonutrients called polyphenols, also found in green tea and grape seeds.

Appendix B

VITAMIN SUPPLEMENT RECOMMENDATIONS

WE'VE SPOKEN ABOUT vitamins and minerals as well as micronutrients. Not all vitamins are equal when it comes to treating blood pressure. These heart-healthy vitamin recommendations may help you
lower your blood pressure.

A Note on Dosages: I have used IU (international units), milligrams, and micrograms in stating specific doses. Not all of the doses
in milligrams are given in IU, since the potency of different vitamins
varies. For example, 100 IU of vitamin A may not be the equivalent of
100 IU of vitamin D.

Vitamin A

You know that eating carrots, rich in vitamin A (beta carotene), prevents vision loss. Vitamin A also cleanses the blood of free radicals and
may even play a role in heart disease prevention.

There is generally no need to take vitamin A supplements, since most
Americans have adequate amounts of vitamin A from diet as well as any
multivitamins that are part of the daily regimen. Also, I would not recommend taking vitamin A supplements due to the lack of return and the
potential toxicity associated with excess. Besides carrots, good sources of
vitamin A include liver, broccoli leaves, pumpkin, collard greens, cantaloupe, eggs, apricots, papayas, mangoes, peas, and winter squash.

Vitamin B/Folic Acid

Folate or folic acid works with vitamin B12 and vitamin C to form red
blood cells. It may even help lower high blood pressure in some peo-

ple. One possible way folic acid lowers blood pressure is by reducing elevated homocysteine levels in people with high blood pressure.

You can easily consume the recommended daily amount of folic acid in your diet by eating beans, peanuts and legumes, citrus fruits, dark green leafy vegetables, poultry, pork, shellfish, and liver. Adequate amounts of folic acid are especially important in some groups such as women of childbearing age.

Vitamin C

Ascorbic acid or vitamin C is an antioxidant that may play a role in fighting cancer. Clinically, vitamin C has been thought to possibly relieve symptoms of high blood pressure, although it has not yet been proven to fight heart disease.

Besides citrus fruits and juices, good food sources of vitamin C include strawberries, sweet red peppers, tomatoes, broccoli, and potatoes.

Vitamin D

A growing body of research suggests that increasing your intake of vitamin D, which regulates the body's metabolic actions and regulates the amount of calcium and phosphorus in the blood, may lower blood pressure. The blood vessels and the heart have large numbers of vitamin D receptors, which indicates that vitamin D plays a role in cardiovascular health.

While I can't definitively say that a vitamin D deficiency contributes to high blood pressure, people with low levels of vitamin D are more likely to develop cardiovascular disease. Studies suggest that low vitamin D levels combined with high blood pressure nearly double the risk of myocardial infarction, stroke, and heart failure.

That said, exposure to sunlight and/or consumption of foods rich in vitamin D is your best bet for your daily dose of vitamin D. During dark or rainy winter months, blood pressure rises as sun exposure diminishes. Fifteen minutes of sun exposure (natural or by means of a sunlamp) every day provide you with a generous dose of vitamin D. Salmon, milk (especially Vitamin D enriched), eggs, mushrooms, tuna, and vitamin D-enriched flour and baked goods are all excellent dietary sources of this vitamin.

Make sure you know how much vitamin D you need, since an excess of vitamin D can cause toxic buildup in the body. For example, people 50 to 70 years old need more than younger counterparts and may also benefit more from supplemental doses with regard to blood pressure.

Vitamin E

Vitamin E (D-alpha tocopherol) is an antioxidant along with vitamins A and C. Though it has been thought that vitamin E may reduce your risk for cancer and heart disease, this does not appear to be the case currently. However, not all vitamin E is created equal. Many nutritionists believe the natural form of vitamin E to be healthier than the synthetic version (DL-alpha tocopherol). Therefore, taking vast quantities of vitamin E capsules (as with any vitamin) is detrimental. Some researchers have suggested that gradually increasing vitamin E dosage lowers blood pressure gradually and safely, but this is yet unproven.

Most Americans get sufficient vitamin E from dietary sources, but people on low-fat diets may need supplementation. There are reports that vitamin E can actually cause an increase in blood pressure if taken in excess. The U.S. Institute of Medicine recommends 1,000 milligrams per day (equivalent to 1,500 IU) as the maximum upper limit dose for supplementary D-alpha tocopherol.

Most adult men and women should consume vitamin E through dietary means, and supplementation is generally not necessary. Good sources of vitamin E include vegetable oils, sesame seeds, sunflower seeds, whole-grain breads, cereals and pastas, nuts, spinach, broccoli, mangoes, kiwifruit, egg yolks, and wheat germ.

Vitamin K

Vitamin K, a fat-soluble vitamin, is better known as potassium. This book has explored its role in regulating blood pressure (see Chapter 3). Some research suggests that vitamin K may be more powerful as an antioxidant and anti-high-blood-pressure micronutrient than vitamin E or even coenzyme Q10. Vitamin K assists in neuron firing, sustains normal heart rate and blood pressure, prevents blood clots, and instigates muscular contractions. Pregnant women may need higher dosages. In addition, some antibiotics may lead to a vitamin

K deficiency. Use caution if you are taking an anticoagulant (anti-blood-clot) medication.

Zinc

Many supplements supposedly formulated to lower blood pressure include zinc. This mineral is an antioxidant that fights cardiovascular disease and eliminates free radicals. It helps maintain the proper levels of vitamin E in the blood, and this helps reduce blood pressur and regulates arterial flow of blood. Zinc may also lower high blood pressure caused by too much cadmium. Not much zinc is needed to keep blood pressure low. Good food sources of zinc are meat, poultry, seafood, eggs, nuts, seeds, and grains.

Selenium

Low levels of selenium are associated with cardiovascular disease, since selenium helps regulate blood flow and cleanses the blood of cadmium, a mineral that increases blood pressure. Selenium acts to cleanse the blood of free radicals and to maintain a healthy heart and blood vessels. You can boost your selenium by consuming Brazil nuts, whole grains, and shellfish.

Phosphorus

Phosphorus combines with other minerals to lower blood pressure. Beware: Too much phosphorus can result in an increase of heart-related deaths in patients who have chronic kidney disease or prior heart disease. Adults ages 70 and over should reduce levels of phosphorus consumption.

Good dietary sources of phosphorus include milk and dairy products, dried peas, beans, and lentils as well as nuts and seeds.

Appendix C

AWAY-FROM-HOME DINING TIPS

Heart-Healthy Dining Tips

- Some menu items and servers go into detail about how the food is prepared. If no details are provided, ask your server about any hidden monounsaturated or saturated fats that the dish may contain.
- Ask about the sodium content of your meal.
- Order a baked potato, steamed vegetables, rice (brown), or pasta instead of the higher-calorie options that are loaded with saturated fat.
- Request salad dressing, sour cream, gravy, and other condiments on the side, or request a mix of balsamic vinegar and olive oil.
- Share an entrée or take home any unused part of your entrée, since most restaurants offer too-generous portion sizes. Look for menus that offer petite, individual, or half portions.
- At self-serve, cafeteria, or buffet restaurants, avoid or limit Worcestershire sauce, pickles, salty barbecue sauce, horseradish, ketchup, and soy sauce (except soy sauce labeled as low-sodium). Ask your server at sit-down restaurants or the order person at fast-food restaurants to hold the ketchup and pickle.
- Choose dishes prepared with lemon, lime, vinegar, herbs, spices, and salt-free seasoning blends.
- Avoid "junk" snacking on the go at stores, kiosks, and food courts. Pack healthy snacks such as unsalted nuts and popcorn,

carrots, cheese sticks, and whole-grain crackers. Even if you grab a latte, you won't be tempted by the high-calorie muffin made with hydrogenated oils.

- Incorporate soy into your dining-out options whenever possible. Many restaurants now have veggie burgers made with soy, or salads garnished with soybeans.
- Opt for meats such as pork prepared in saucy marinades, which reduce unhealthy compounds called cholesterol oxidization products.

Some Lower-Sodium Restaurant Options*

- Charbroiler Express makes a burger and fries with no sodium.
- Fuddrucker's makes a burger and fries with no sodium.
- Golden Corral has menus with nutritional breakdowns; call ahead for no sodium.
- In-N-Out Burger (California, Nevada, Utah) gives you the option to order burger patties without sodium.
- At McCormick and Schmick's Seafood Restaurants, call ahead to request no sodium.
- Max's Opera Café will serve vegetables and vegetarian entrées with no salt or sauces, and will grill or broil entreés on request.
- At Outback Steakhouse locations, waiters will accommodate dietary restrictions and tell you that baked potatoes usually come with salt and butter on the outside.
- The Red Robin chain features the Protein Burger Lettuce Wrap (no sodium). You can request no salt on steak fries.

*Tips adapted from http://www.megaheart.com/restaurants.html. (Remember that although these items are lower in sodium, they aren't necessarily "heart healthy.")

Appendix D

OVERCOMING ADDICTIONS TO FOOD, ALCOHOL, TOBACCO, AND DRUGS

Food

AS WE'VE SAID, losing weight and eating healthy are two of the most powerful weapons to bring down high blood pressure. However, some people may have an addiction to food that renders them unable to stop eating. Food addicts:

- Think about food constantly
- Try to stop eating without success
- Attempt one diet plan after another and fail
- Binge and then vomit or use laxatives to purge the food
- Binge without vomiting
- Eat large quantities of food in private
- Eat when they're not hungry
- Feel less and less satisfied with food
- Nibble all day long and thus develop a weight problem
- Eat to escape uncomfortable feelings
- Hide or hoard food
- Fast or starve themselves in order to lose weight
- Obsessively exercise to lose weight
- Obsessively compare calories burned to calories eaten
- Feel ashamed or guilty after eating

These are all symptoms of eating disorders. No one knows what causes eating disorders—they may develop from anxiety, trauma, a desire to control one's life. What we do know is that they have disastrous effects on life and health.

If you are a food addict, it's important to seek treatment immediately. As with major addictions, treatment may take any or all of the forms below:

- Counseling to change your thoughts and behaviors, to modify eating habits and substitute healthy ones for unhealthy ones
- Twelve-step programs or support groups
- Nutrition counseling
- Medication
- Alternative health practices such as yoga, meditation, and t'ai chi

Unlike smoking, or alcohol or illicit drugs, food is necessary for life. A changed attitude toward food is vital for the success of your recovery. Some tips:

- Instead of eating when you are stressed or whenever your thoughts or feelings trigger the urge, take a brisk walk. Studies show that the activity produces the same pleasurable feelings as eating a bowl of candy.
- Write down the triggers that cause you to overeat, and carry that list with you. Recognize the situations that cause you to overeat, and avoid them if at all possible.
- Distract yourself until the compulsion to eat passes.
- Drink at least 64 ounces of water per day, which helps you feel full.

For help, visit:

Food Addicts in Recovery Anonymous: http://www.foodaddicts.org
Overeaters Anonymous: http://www.oa.org/index.htm

Alcohol

People deny alcoholism every day. However, if you have taken the step toward admitting you might have a problem, ask yourself the following questions:

- Have you tried to reduce your drinking?
- Have you felt bad about drinking?
- Have you been annoyed by another person's criticism of your drinking?
- Do you drink in the morning to steady your nerves or cure a hangover?
- Do you have problems with a job, your family, or the law?
- Do you drive under the influence of alcohol?
- Do you crave a drink, or are you unable to stop or limit drinking?
- Do you need greater amounts of alcohol to feel the same effect?
- Does your drinking continue even though it causes or worsens your high blood pressure?

If you answered yes to more than two of these questions, you are not in denial. You genuinely recognize you may have a problem. You know that in addition to the other devastating consequences of alcohol abuse, you are driving up your blood pressure.

You may be afraid of the withdrawal symptoms in addition to craving the chemical dependency. Withdrawal symptoms include:

- Nausea
- Sweating
- Shaking
- Anxiety
- Increased blood pressure
- Seizures (delirium tremens, "DTs")

Your doctor can help you withdraw from alcohol safely if you desire to change. This could require hospitalization in a detoxification center. The detoxification center staff will carefully monitor you for side effects. You may need medication while you are undergoing detoxification.

Some medications may reduce alcohol craving. This is important because most professionals who treat alcoholism believe *abstinence is the only effective prevention*.

The medication and abstinence can work in conjunction with therapy and counseling that will help you recognize alcohol's dangers. Therapy raises awareness of underlying issues and lifestyles that promote drinking. In therapy, you work to improve coping skills and learn other ways of dealing with stress or pain (such as the de-stressing techniques in Chapter 8 of this book). Also, Alcoholics Anonymous or AA and/or other addiction and recovery groups help many people to stop drinking and stay sober.

Many people who enter treatment for alcohol abuse and dependency make sobriety a way of life. They practice prevention, which means they:

- Socialize without alcohol.
- Avoid going to bars.
- Do not keep alcohol in the home.
- Avoid situations and people that encourage drinking.
- Make new nondrinking friends.
- Do fun things that do not involve alcohol.
- Avoid reaching for a drink when stressed or upset.
- Limit alcohol intake to a moderate level.
  - Moderate is two or fewer drinks per day for men and one or fewer for women and older adults.
  - A 12-ounce bottle of beer, a five-ounce glass of wine, or 1.5 ounces of liquor is considered one drink.

You can make these changes to bring down your blood pressure and boost your quality of life. For more information and help, visit Alcoholics Anonymous, http://www.alcoholics-anonymous.org, as well as the National Council on Alcoholism and Drug Dependence, http://www.ncadd.org.

Tobacco

We spoke about the effect smoking has on blood pressure. For many people, quitting smoking is difficult. Nicotine is one of the most addictive drugs known. When you combine this chemical with the flavor of tobacco smoke and the oral satisfaction of a cigarette, you get an addiction to tobacco that is very difficult to break.

Tobacco addiction occurs when the use of tobacco harms a person's health or social functioning, or when a person becomes dependent on tobacco. Tobacco may be consumed in the form of cigarettes; smokeless tobacco products (e.g., snuff, chewing tobacco); cigars; or pipes.

Symptoms of and health problems related to tobacco abuse include:

- Hyperglycemia (abnormally high blood sugar level)
- Withdrawal: nervousness, headache, irritability, cravings, sleep disturbances, difficulty concentrating or paying attention
- Spikes in blood pressure, respiration, and heart rate
- Smoker's cough
- Heart disease
- Stroke
- Emphysema
- Throat cancer
- Chronic obstructive pulmonary disease
- Pregnancy complications and miscarriage
- Chronic bronchitis

These conditions and symptoms may not in themselves indicate tobacco addiction and abuse. However, if you have a problem, medications may help people quit smoking by easing symptoms of nicotine withdrawal and may block the effects of nicotine if people resume smoking. Behavior modification therapy, including counseling and hypnosis, can help you curb the urge to smoke in stressful situations or at times when you normally light up. (Hypnotherapy experts note that quitting smoking and losing weight are the two main services hypnotherapy patients want.)

Nicotine replacement therapy such as patches, gums, nasal sprays, and inhalers can help relieve the unpleasant nicotine withdrawal symptoms.

If you smoke, here are some strategies that may help you quit smoking.

- Set a quit date. Write it on your calendar and create electronic reminders.
- Change to a lower-tar brand or a brand you find less appealing or even distasteful. Do this two weeks before your quit date.
- Smoke only half of each cigarette.
- Decide you'll smoke at different times of the day than you normally do—one hour before you usually light up, for example.
- Set a limit on how many cigarettes you'll smoke, and for each cigarette beyond that limit, give a dollar to your favorite charity.

- Change your eating habits—drink more milk, for example, which for many people seems incompatible with smoking. Drink a glass of juice for energy instead of smoking a cigarette.
- Don't empty your ashtrays. Let the smell and sight remind you how much you smoke.
- Catch yourself before you light up out of habit.
- Put the cigarettes in a location where you can't easily get to them or reach them. Don't carry them with you. Force yourself to think about smoking, which will give you time to choose not to smoke.
- Buy cigarettes one pack at a time (and watch the cost add up).
- Look in a mirror each time you smoke. The sight may make you change your mind.
- Smoke alone if you usually smoke with others, and focus your attention on the negative aspects of smoking. Smoke in situations you find less than pleasant. This will make you associate smoking with discomfort.
- Take quitting one day at a time—tell yourself you won't smoke today, and then don't.
- Practice going without cigarettes, pipes, cigars, or whatever your tobacco delivery device is.
- Collect all your cigarette butts in one economy-size glass container as a visual reminder of the filth made by smoking.
- Clean or dry-clean your clothes to get rid of the tobacco smell and enjoy the clean scent afterward.
- On the day you quit, go for a bike ride, take a walk, or exercise to get a natural high.
- Spend time with nonsmoking friends and family and ask for their support on your quit date as well as the first few days and weeks.
- Make a list of gifts you'd like to buy for yourself or a loved one, vacations you'd like to take, et cetera. Estimate the cost in terms of packs of cigarettes, and put the money you would have spent aside to buy what you want.
- Buy yourself a treat or something special to celebrate.
- Have your teeth cleaned and whitened to get rid of tobacco stains. Take an "after" photo if possible. Notice how nice your teeth look and resolve to keep them that way.
- Enjoy the feeling of breathing fully and calmly.

- Enjoy how healthy and appealing your house, car, and clothes smell without cigarettes.
- After you quit, spend as much free time as possible in smoke-free locations such as museums, art galleries, libraries, churches, department stores, and theaters.
- Carry a pencil, phone/iPod, button, electronic gadget, or other substitute to play with instead of a cigarette.
- Buy yourself flowers—the aroma will comfort you. Air out your home and office with plants.
- Don't ask for a match for your cigarette to strike up a conversation.
- Drink lots of fluids, especially water and fruit juice.

For more information and help visit:

American Lung Association, http://www.lungusa.org
CDC—Tobacco Information and Prevention Source (TIPS), http://www.cdc.gov/tobacco/index.htm
National Cancer Institute, http://smokefree.gov
U.S. Department of Health and Human Services, 1-800 Quit-Now, http://1800quitnow.cancer.gov

Illicit Drugs/Prescription Drugs

Drug abuse is a disease characterized by continued misuse of drugs even when faced with drug-related job, legal, health, or family difficulties.

Here are some signs of drug abuse to be aware of:

- Repeated work, school, or home problems due to drug use
- Continued use of drugs even though it means risking physical safety
- Recurring trouble with the law related to drug use, including impaired driving
- Continuing to use drugs despite drug-related problems in personal relationships

Drug abuse progresses to drug dependence, which refers to long-term, compulsive drug use. The user may make attempts to stop but repeatedly return to drugs. Drug dependence also means that your body has begun to require the drug in higher doses to avoid withdrawal symptoms. Symptoms of drug dependence include the following:

- Craving for drugs
- Inability to stop or limit drug use
- Increased tolerance, taking greater amounts to feel the same effect
- Withdrawal symptoms when the drug is stopped
- Significant amounts of time trying to acquire drugs and recover from their effects
- Giving up activities to use drugs or recover from the effects
- Continuing drug use even when it causes or worsens health and/ or psychological problems

The most commonly abused substances include:

- Cocaine
- Heroin
- Morphine
- LSD
- Marijuana
- Sedatives
- Speed, methamphetamine, "crystal meth" (an instantly addictive drug that devastates body and mind)
- PCP
- Ecstasy
- GHB
- Ketamine
- Steroids
- Inhalants
- Legal drugs that are used improperly or without a prescription, such as narcotic painkillers, amphetamines, sleeping pills, and antianxiety and antidepressant medications

Drug abuse and use of illicit drugs may have significant impact on your blood pressure and may even interfere with blood pressure medications.

As with treatment for alcohol abuse, medication, counseling, and self-help organizations such as Narcotics Anonymous and Cocaine Anonymous are important steps in becoming drug-free.

You can overcome drug addiction by taking other preventive steps:

- Learn about risks related to drug use.
- Do not spend time with people who are using illegal drugs.
- Learn coping skills to handle peer pressure and stress.
- Seek counseling for anxiety, depression, and other mental health problems.

For more information and help, you may want to visit:

Narcotics Anonymous, http://www.na.org
National Institute on Drug Abuse, http://www.nida.nih.gov
MEDLINE Prescription Drug Abuse Information: http://www.nlm
   .nih.gov/medlineplus/prescriptiondrugabuse.html
Cocaine Anonymous, http://www.ca.org
Heroin Anonymous, http://www.heroin-anonymous.org
Marijuana Anonymous, http://www.marijuana-anonymous.org
The Meth Project, http://notevenonce.com

Appendix E

APPROVED HEALTH ORGANIZATIONS

I WOULD LIKE TO recognize and thank some extraordinary organizations that help improve health and quality of life. Although this list is certainly not all-inclusive, it gives me great pleasure to include the following in a selected list.

- American Cancer Society
- American Heart Association
- Atlas Ergonomics, Inc.
- Centers for Disease Control and Prevention
- Cooper Aerobics Center
- Exan Wellness
- GlaxoSmithKline
- Gojo, Inc.
- Integrated Benefits Institute
- National Center for Health Statistics
- Nurtur Health
- Pfizer
- Weight Watchers
- YMCA

INDEX

acupuncture, 205
adrenal glands, 245
adrenaline, 141, 214
African Americans, 8, 10, 16
Aggressive Standards for Advancement of Medical Instruments, 6
aging: blood pressure and, 7; exercise and, 19, 141–42; medication and, 194
Alaska Natives, 8–9
alcohol addiction, 266–68
alcohol consumption, 9, 250–51
aldosteronism, 245
Almond-Crusted Tilapia, 119
alpha blockers, 184
alternative therapies: acupuncture, 205; amino acids, 201–2; bath therapy, 201; bitter orange, 207–8; coenzyme Q10, 204; dark chocolate, 202; dietary supplements, 198–99, 259–62; DMAE (dimethylaminoethanol), 207–9; effective, 197–203; ephedra and related products, 206–7; examples of, 197; fish oil, 199; future and experimental, 208–9; gene therapy/genomics, 208–9; grape juice, 203; green tea, 203; hawthorn, 204; licorice, 206; má huáng, 206–7; massage, 201, 205–6;

mineral supplements, 262; mud baths, 204; nutrigenomics, 209; omega-3 fatty acids, 199, 258; pseudoephedrine, 206–7; reflexology, 205–6; resveratrol, 203; secondary high blood pressure and, 246; stem cell treatments, 209–10; stevia, 201–2; superfoods, 255–58; tetrandrine, 206; unproven, 203–6; unsafe, 206–8; vitamin supplements, 259–62; yoga, qigong, t'ai chi, 199–201; yohimbe/yohimbine, 206
ambulatory blood pressure monitoring (ABPM), 239
American Heart Association, 2, 9
amino acids, 201–2
aneurysms, 253
anger, repressed, 10, 215–17
angiotensin-converting enzyme (ACE), 22
angiotensin-converting enzyme (ACE) inhibitors, 178, 188–89, 203
angiotensin-II receptor antagonists (ARBs), 178–79
angiotensin inhibitors, 189
aorta, coarctation of the, 246
appetizer recipes, 56–66
apples, 255–56
arthritis, 146–52

complementary alternative medicine (CAM), 198, 210–11. *See also* alternative therapies

contraceptive use, 9

cooking tips, 38–41, 52. *See also* recipes

Corn Chowder, 90

cottage cheese, 258

Council on Physical Fitness and Sports, 145–46

Crab and Roasted Corn Soup, 93

Cranberry Salad, 75

crash diets, 23

C-reactive protein (CRP), 24–25, 45, 249

Crispy Edamame, 101

Cuban Black Bean Soup, 89

Cucumber Couscous Salad, 78

cupuaçu, 258

Curtido Cabbage Salvadore, 59

Cushing's syndrome, 245

dairy products, 47–48, 258

DASH diet (Dietary Approaches to Stop Hypertension), 30–31, 173

death, high blood pressure-related, 8, 12, 14, 16

dessert recipes, 125–30

diabetic nephropathy, 244

diastolic pressure, 2, 241

diet: alternative therapies, 202–3; beverages, 42–43, 49–50; blood pressure and, 163–67; calcium in, 47; carbohydrates in, 43–44; dark chocolate, including in, 202; dining away from home, tips for, 263–64; eliminating 100 calories, 166; exercise and, 51; fiber in, 40; food addictions, 265–66; goals for changes in, 27; micronutrients, 33–37; portion size control, 25–26; sodium

and, 27–30; superfoods, 255–58; time-saving tips, 52; vegetarian, 250. *See also* grocery, shopping for; recipes

dietary supplements, 198–99, 259–62

diets, specific: DASH diet (Dietary Approaches to Stop Hypertension), 30–31; low-carbohydrate, 43–44; Optimum Health Low-Sodium, 30–31; very-high-protein, 45

dining away from home, tips for, 263–64

diuretics, 182–83, 189–90

DMAE (dimethylaminoethanol), 207–9

doctor visits. *See* physicians

drug abuse, 10, 246, 271–73

eating disorders, 265–66

eggs, recipes with, 107

egg whites, 255

emotion, effect on blood pressure, 10, 215–17, 229–30

encephalopathy (disease of the brain), 5

English Muffin Bread, 74

entrées, recipes for, 104–20

environmental factors for high blood pressure, 9–10

ephedra/ephedrine/pseudoephedrine and related products, 206–7

erectile dysfunction, 10–12, 247–48

essential high blood pressure. *See* primary high blood pressure

exercise: aerobic, 137, 140, 144, 149–52; aging and, 19, 141–42; anaerobic, 145–46; benefits of, 17–18, 139–42, 148, 164; beta-blockers and, 180; creative, 138,

impotence, 10–12, 247–48
insulin resistance/sensitivity, 141, 220, 250
insurance, health, 16
Island-Style Grilling Marinade, 122

Joint National Committee on Prevention, Detection Evaluation and Treatment of High Blood Pressure (JNC 6) Risk Stratification System, 175–77
Joint National Committee on Prevention, Detection Evaluation and Treatment of High Blood Pressure (JNC 7) report, 3, 5, 173–74

"Keeping It Simple" approach, 46
kidney disease/failure, 5, 8, 15, 244–45
kola nut, 207

LDL (bad cholesterol), 45
legumes. *See* beans and legumes, recipes with
Lemon Tarragon Chicken, 109
Lentil Soup, 92
licorice, 206
lifestyle choices, 9–10
Louisiana-Style Shrimp Creole, 113
low blood pressure, 240–42
low-carbohydrate diets, 43–44

magnesium, 33–37
má huáng, 206–7
Maple Crisp Bars, 128
marinades, seasonings, and rubs, 121–24
massage, 201, 205–6, 223
meat, recipes with: *Asian Pork-Fried Rice*, 112; *Herb-Marinated*

Lamb Chops, 117; *Spicy and Sweet Meatballs*, 58
medication: alpha blockers, 184; alternative therapies to avoid combining with, 206–8; angiotensin-converting enzyme inhibitors, 178, 188–89; angiotensin-II receptor antagonists, 178–79; angiotensin inhibitors, 189; beta-blockers, 179–80, 189–90; calcium antagonists, 180–82; calcium channel blockers, 180–82, 188–90; combination therapies, 185–91; costs, 194; diuretics, 182–83, 189–90; effectiveness factors, 14; eliminating the need for, 14; generics, 194; JNC 6 Risk Stratification System, 175–77; JNC 7 recommendations, 173–75; misconceptions about, 193; nitroglycerin/nitrate vasodilators, 184–85; noncompliance statistics, 16; prescription, abusing, 271–73; reducing need for, 177, 193; refills, 192–93; risks of high blood pressure from, 10, 246; stopping, 193–94; TAKE guidelines, 191–93. *See also* alternative therapies
meditation, 230–32
Mediterranean Orzo Pasta, 97
Mediterranean Pasta Salad, 76
men, risk of high blood pressure in, 7, 12, 16, 247–48
menopause, 246–47
Mexican Pozole, 60
migraine headaches, 251–52
mindfulness, 160
mineral supplements, 262
Minestrone, 85

qigong, 199–201, 230–32
quinoa, 257

race, effect on high blood pressure,
     8–9, 16, 248
Raspberry Streusel Muffins, 68
recipes: appetizers, 56–66; bread,
     67–74; cooking tips, 38–41,
     52; desserts, 125–30; entrées,
     104–20; marinades, seasonings,
     and rubs, 121–24; salads, 75–84;
     soups, 85–93; vegetables/side
     dishes, 94–103. *See also* diet
reflexology, 205–6
Refreshing Orange-Pineapple Sherbet,
     130
resveratrol, 203
rice, recipes with: *Asian Pork-Fried
     Rice*, 112; *Tasty Rice Pudding*, 129
rice and pasta, 40–41
Roasted Acorn Squash, 100
Roasted Red Pepper Hummus, 64
Roasted Sweet Potatoes, 99
Roasted Vegetable Salad, 77
Roberts, William, 18

salads and salad dressing, 37–38,
     75–84
Salmon Almondine, 108
salt sensitivity, 9–10
San Francisco Cioppino, 87–88
Sautéed Calamari, 120
scheduling: blood pressure
     screenings, 14; checkups, 14, 194,
     239–40; exercise, 167; for stress
     reduction, 222–23, 226–27
Schwarzenegger, Arnold, 145–46
seafood, recipes with: *Crab and
     Roasted Corn Soup*, 93; *Louisiana-
     Style Shrimp Creole*, 113; *San
     Francisco Cioppino*, 87–88; *Sautéed
     Calamari*, 120; *Seared Garlic*

Scallops, 114; *Spanish Chicken
     and Shrimp Paella*, 110; *Spicy
     Marinated Shrimp Bowl*, 61
Seared Garlic Scallops, 114
secondary high blood pressure, 9,
     243–46
selenium, 262
sexual performance, 10–12, 247–48
sleep apnea, 220, 246
sleep deprivation, 219–20
smoking, 9, 223, 268–71
social networks and stress, 223, 226,
     230
sodium consumption, 9–10
sodium content in food, 27–30
soups and soup recipes, 49, 85–93
soy, 257
Spanish Chicken and Shrimp Paella,
     110
spices. *See* herbs and spices
Spicy and Sweet Meatballs, 58
Spicy Marinated Shrimp Bowl, 61
Spicy Santa Fe Chicken Fajitas, 111
Spinach Lasagna, 105–6
spirituality and stress reduction,
     220–22
stem cell therapy, 209–10
stevia, 201–2
stress journal, 224
stress reduction: deep breathing
     for, 222; emotional habits to
     practice, 229–30; exercise for,
     218–19; faith and spirituality
     for, 220–22; financial, 223,
     227–28; introduction to, 213–14;
     Lorenzo's story, 215–17; massage
     for, 201, 205–6; mindful exercise
     for, 160, 199–201, 230–32; saying
     "no" and, 224–27; sleep and,
     219–20; suggestions for, 222–24
stress response, 214–15
stroke, 1–2, 8, 15

Summer Corn and Tomato Salad, 82
Summer Vegetable Ratatouille, 102
superfoods, 255–58
systolic pressure, 2, 241

Tabbouleh, 103
t'ai chi, 199–201, 230–32
TAKE guidelines, 191–93
Tasty Rice Pudding, 129
tea, green, 203
tetrandrine (Stephania tetrandra), 206
thyroid glands, 245
thyroid hormones, 207
tobacco, 268–71
travel: dining away from home, tips for, 263–64; exercise on-the-go, 153–54
turkey, recipes with: Polynesian Turkey Kabobs, 104; Turkey Soup with Barley, 86
Turkey Soup with Barley, 86

Vaughan, Bill, 17
Vegetable-Flounder Bake, 115
Vegetable Orzo Primavera, 118
vegetable recipes, 94–103
vegetables, 37–39, 256
vegetables, recipes with: Autumn Succotash, 96; Broccoli-Cauliflower-Carrot Bake, 98; Caribbean Sweet Potato Salad, 81; Corn Chowder, 90; Crab and Roasted Corn Soup, 93; Crispy Edamame, 101; Cucumber Couscous Salad, 78; Curtido Cabbage Salvadore, 59; Gazpacho, 65; Glazed Parsnip Salad with Pecans, 84; Green Beans with Slivered Almonds, Garlic, and Basil, 94; Mexican Pozole, 60; Minestrone, 85; New Orleans Chicken Gumbo

with Okra, 91; Pan-Fried Yucca, 63; Pecan and Avocado Salad, 83; Roasted Acorn Squash, 100; Roasted Sweet Potatoes, 99; Roasted Vegetable Salad, 77; Spinach Lasagna, 105–6; Summer Corn and Tomato Salad, 82; Summer Vegetable Ratatouille, 102; Vegetable-Flounder Bake, 115; Vegetable Orzo Primavera, 118; Zucchini Bread, 69
vegetarianism, 250
vitamin supplements, 259–62
volunteering, 223–24

waist size, 24, 249–50
weight loss: basics of, 22–23, 25; benefits of, 21–22, 165; goals for, 26–27, 165–66; motivation, maintaining for, 164–65; portion size control for, 25–26; reasonable goals for, 25; recommendations, 25; success factors, 26; without exercise, 164
Wesley, John, 224
Whole Wheat Popovers, 70
wine, red, 203
women, risk of high blood pressure in, 7, 8, 16, 40, 219
women and high blood pressure, 246–48
Wooden, John, 224
workplace: exercise in the, 152–54, 167; saying no in the, 226

yerba mate, 207
yoga, 199–201, 230–32
yohimbe/yohimbine, 206
young adults, 8

zinc, 262
Zucchini Bread, 69